Simulation Training in Laparoscopy and Robotic Surgery

D1486122

Hitendra R.H. Patel • Jean V. Joseph

Editors

Simulation Training in Laparoscopy and Robotic Surgery

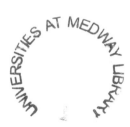

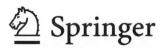 Springer

Editors
Hitendra R.H. Patel, MD, PhD
Department of Urology and Endocrine
Surgery, University Hospital North Norway
Tromsø
Norway

Jean V. Joseph, M.D., MBA
Department of Urology
University of Rochester Medical Center for
Robotic Surgery and Innovation
Rochester
New York
USA

ISBN 978-1-4471-2929-5   ISBN 978-1-4471-2930-1   (eBook)
DOI 10.1007/978-1-4471-2930-1
Springer London Heidelberg New York Dordrecht

Library of Congress Control Number: 2012936654

© Springer-Verlag London 2012

To my wife Venita for all her support over the last 15 years.

Foreword

The editors are commended for bringing together the very latest ideas and evidence on simulation training in laparoscopic and robotic surgery from pre-eminent authors in this emerging field. The book is very well structured, with each chapter commencing with an abstract and key words, whilst a key points section alerts as to what the reader might expect to learn. It is very well referenced with citations of traditional printed publications and also some to some useful websites.

The introduction reminds us of the countless lives saved by the introduction of basic checklists and teamwork training across the aviation industry, which has become an examplar for safe working practice. Subsequent chapters cover human factors in general. The importance of non-technical surgical skills and the current state of laparoscopic, robotic and minimally invasive surgery training. The role of virtual reality simulation is discussed, with contributions on how the addition of binocular 3D vision and haptics increases fidelity. Many advances in surgery result from lessons learned on battlefields, and novel ideas on trauma simulation from the military are shared. Finally the value of distance learning, multimedia, e-learning and telementoring is scrutinised, something that is particularly appropriate for 'generation Z' who are about to enter surgical training.

This book is a great read and will bring surgeons of any specialty up to date on surgical simulation in general, particularly in laparoscopic and robotic surgery. The Joint Committee on Surgical Training, representing the four UK and Irish Surgical Royal Colleges, is currently mapping the requirements for simulation within the Intercollegiate Surgical Curriculum Programme for trainees. The Colleges and a variety of other educational providers are working hard to provide simulation courses to keep up with new technological developments in this area. This book assists with that effort by providing ample evidence of emerging knowledge and pedagogy to support the role of simulation training in surgery. Simulation has become a vital part of surgical training with "see one, do one" being replaced by "sim many before doing one (for real)", and it is now also beginning to take its place within selection and assessment procedures. I heartily recommend this book to today's generation of trainers and trainees.

England   Professor Mike Larvin

Preface

What would the surgical experience be like if every surgeon routinely goes through a warm-up period with the surgical team before embarking on a surgical procedure, similar to what athletes and musicians do prior to performing? One can only speculate on the value of such exercise on the harmony of the operating theater, the surgeon's comfort with the procedure, the surgical outcome, and ultimately the overall patient experience.

In the quest to deliver the best and safest care, upholding the oath to do "no harm," our objective remains to limit the impact of surgical intervention and eliminate variables, which by definition can impact the surgical care we deliver. Simulation-based training, which is heavily used in a number of nonmedical disciplines, promises to be a paradigm shift in medicine and surgery, as its value in medical or surgical education comes to the fore. Simulation offers a platform where a surgeon, or care team, can actually rehearse, learn, improve, or maintain their skills in a safe and stress-free environment.

The aim of our book is to allow anyone with an interest in training or education within surgery, an opportunity to understand the subject. The latest evolution in surgery has been minimally invasive surgery, thus the emphasis in the book has taken examples from this field, notably the greatest advance of robotic surgery.

The flow of the book takes the reader through the art of educating a surgeon using a variety of techniques from Queen Mary University of London to Imperial College London. A cutting-edge chapter on trauma and simulation learning points from the 7/7 London bombings shows a real insight into how important training is for those thankfully rare moments. This highlights the value of education with simulation.

We then traveled through Europe to understand the historical aspects of training in minimally invasive surgery, by an expert surgical innovator of the modern generation (University of Tuebingen). History generally shows that nothing is actually new. Often packaging changes, but the elemental facts remain unchanged. Simulation with modern technology has often been thought of as technology based, such as computer simulators. The University of Indiana has completed a study using a robotic training device which has become the fastest selling training system of its kind in the world. However, when it was being designed, the very process of design is a form of simulation and learning.

This led to the important aspect of understanding where simulation training is performed at the highest level – the airline industry. Checklist for surgery via the World Health Organization is now mandatory in many hospitals across the globe; however, the emphasis on team training in the clinical setting (again a powerful human simulation) is sparse. The nontechnical aspects of this type of training are elegantly brought to the reader from the University of North Norway.

An international telemedical center at the University of North Norway contributes aspects related to continuous learning through simulation and importantly mentoring through this type of initiation learning (or proctoring). This is an exciting and expanding subject, which has stimulated a significant advance in recent months. Of particular interest is the portable learning system for surgeons or their teams to use as an "aide memoir" or even as a core-learning tool. Ultimately, we think this latest tool will be the future way of teaching and learning for both doctor and patient.

Tromsø, Norway   Hitendra R.H. Patel
Rochester, NY   Jean V. Joseph

Acknowledgement

To the wonderful support from the Springer team.

Contents

Contributors

Waleed Al-Singary, Dip(Urol), MPhil, FEB(Urol), FRCS(Urol)
Western Sussex Hospital NHS Trust, Sussex Medical Center,
Worthing, West Sussex, Brighton, UK

Llandough Hospital, Cardiff, UK

Nottingham City Hospital, Nottingham, UK

Benenden Hospital, Kent, UK

Sonal Arora, B.Sc.(hons), MBBS, MRCS Departments of Surgery and Cancer,
Imperial College, London, UK

Knut Magne Augestad, M.D. Norwegian Center of Telemedicine,
University Hospital North Norway, Tromsø, Norway

Johan G. Bellika, Ph.D. Medical Informatics & Telemedicine Group,
Department of Computer Science, University of Tromsø, Tromsø, Norway

Amina A. Bouhelal, MBBS, M.Sc. London Surgical Academy, Cancer Institute,
Barts and The London School of Medicine and Dentistry, London, UK

Taridzo Chomutare, M.Sc. Norwegian Centre for Integrated Care
& Telemedicine, University Hospital of North Norway, Tromsø, Norway

Conor P. Delaney, MB, MCh, Ph.D., FRCSI, FACS, FASCRS Division
of Colorectal Surgery, Department of Surgery, University Hospitals Case Medical
Center, Case Western Reserve University, Cleveland, OH, USA

Simon S. Fleming, MBBS(Lond), MRCS(Eng), M.Sc.(Surg) Queen Mary
University of London, London, UK

Barts & The London Medical School and NHS Trust, London, Great Britain, UK

Thomas Frede, M.D. Department of Urology, Helios Kliniken,
Muellheim, Germany

Marcel Hruza, M.D. Department of Urology, SLK-Kliniken Heilbronn GmbH, Heilbronn, Germany

Roger Kneebone, Ph.D., FRCS, FrCGP Departments of Surgery and Cancer, Imperial College, London, UK

Narinderjit Singh Kullar, MBBS, M.Sc.(MedEd), MRCS Department of Urology and Endocrine Surgery, University Hospital North Norway, Breivika, Tromsø, Norway

Rolv-Ole Lindsetmo, M.D., Ph.D., MPH Department of Gastrointestinal Surgery, University Hospital North Norway, Tromsø, Norway

Steven M. Lucas, M.D. Department of Urology, Indiana University, Indianapolis, IN, USA

Salvatore Micali, M.D. Policlinico de Modena, University of Modena & Reggio Emilia, Modena, Italy

Mobile Medical Mentor (M3) Project Group

Stig Müller, M.D., Ph.D. Department of Urology and Endocrine Surgery, University Hospital North Norway, Breivika, Tromsø, Norway

Bijendra Patel, MBBS, MS, FRCS(Ed), FRCS(Gen.Surg) Department of Upper GI Surgery, Barts Cancer Institute and Royal London Hospital, Queen Mary University of London, Barbican, London, UK

Hitendra R.H. Patel, MD, PhD Department of Urology and Endocrine Surgery, University Hospital North Norway, Breivika, Tromsø, Norway

Jens J. Rassweiler, M.D. Department of Urology, SLK-Kliniken Heilbronn GmbH, Heilbronn, Germany

John-Joe Reilly, B.Sc.(Hons), GiBiol, Ph.D., DIC, BMedSci(Hons), BM, BS Academic Department of Military Surgery and Trauma, Royal Centre for Defense Medicine, University Hospital Birmingham, Birmingham, UK

Chandru P. Sundaram, M.D. Department of Urology, Indiana University, Indianapolis, IN, USA

Shabnam Undre, MBBS, FRCS, Ph.D. Departments of Surgery and Cancer, Imperial College, London, UK

Andrius Budrionis, M.Sc. Norwegian Centre for Integrated Care and Telemedicine, Tromsø, Norway

Department of Computer Science, North Carolina State University, USA

Chapter 1
Lessons Learned from the Aviation Industry: Surgical Checklists

Stig Müller and Hitendra R.H. Patel

Abstract Checklists are the foundation for safety and quality control in the aviation industry. The concept developed from a disaster in 1935 and to date checklists are a dynamic tool within aviation and aircraft maintenance, regularly audited and adjusted to prevent avoidable error or accidents. Other high-risk industries such as nuclear and oil drilling industries have adapted the checklist principle as a means to improve safety. The recent introduction of the WHO checklist for safe surgery has demonstrated a reduction in perioperative mortality and morbidity and has led to an implementation on a grand scale around the world. The checklist principle though is not novel to health care, many hospitals have used preoperative checklists for years. Critics have therefore dismissed the WHO checklist as "the emperor's new clothes." However, the initial results of the WHO checklist should encourage surgeons to implement checklists as a tool for quality control toward safety-oriented health care.

Keywords WHO checklist • Safe surgery • Boeing B-17 • Aviation training Quality control

> **Key Points**
> - The original checklist principle evolved from disaster.
> - The use of the original checklist turned a faulty prototype into a great success.
> - Checklists can be utilized in training.

S. Müller, M.D., Ph.D. • H.R.H. Patel, MD, PhD (✉)
Department of Urology and Endocrine Surgery, University Hospital North Norway,
Breivika, Tromsø N-9038, Norway
e-mail: hrhpatel@hotmail.com

H.R.H. Patel, J.V. Joseph (eds.), *Simulation Training in Laparoscopy and Robotic Surgery*,   1
DOI 10.1007/978-1-4471-2930-1_1, © Springer-Verlag London 2012

- Reaction patterns in emergency medicine are improved by checklists.
- Task saturation provokes human error.
- Checklists are a tool for quality control.
- The checklist principle is already in use in some areas of medicine.
- Checklists can improve the quality of care in surgery by avoiding human error.
- The WHO checklist improves communication and team factors.
- Overworking checklists can be detrimental and counterproductive to patient safety.

In 1935, the US Army Air Corps was in the final phase of evaluating aircraft specified as heavy bomber aircraft. Boeing had submitted a prototype, the model 299. The aircraft outclassed its competitors in the preliminary evaluations, and the test flights were considered a formality. The test flight took place on October 30, 1935 on Wright Field, Dayton, Ohio.

Shortly after an uneventful takeoff, the aircraft stalled, turned on one wing, fell, and bursted into flames on impact. The test pilots were rescued from the wreckage but later died from their injuries. What had gone wrong? The following investigation concluded that human error had been the cause for the disaster. The pilot, unfamiliar with the prototype and flying it for the first time, neglected to release the elevator lock (elevators control the pitch of the aircraft). This human error led to the uncontrolled ditch. Interestingly, the chief test pilot of Boeing and a Boeing technician were accompanying the test flight, yet the crash was not prevented. Critics labeled the prototype as "too much airplane to fly for one man." Boeing did not receive the main contract, but due to outstanding preliminary results, the Army ordered 12 aircraft. These were delivered to the 2nd Bombardment Group at Langley Field, Virginia, by August 1937. All operations involving the aircraft were closely monitored by Boeing, Congress, and the War Department. Knowing of the cause of the test flight accident, pilots discussed a means of "making sure everything is done and nothing is overlooked." The concept of the pilot's checklist evolved. The initial concept already distinguished checklists for the different phases of a flight from takeoff to after landing. Importantly, these checklists were first implemented on these aircraft, and the error leading to the crash during test flight never occurred again. In fact, the 12 aircraft managed to fly 1.8 million miles without a serious accident. The prototype was later named the B-17, the *Flying Fortress*, and was in military and commercial use until the late 1960s [1].

Seventy-five years later, checklists are the foundation of quality assurance and safety in the airline industry as they are applied in flight operations, aircraft maintenance, as well as human factor training [2].

The surgical checklist has recently been introduced in the course of the World Health Organization (WHO) guidelines for safer surgery. In a global multicenter study, the implementation of the checklist reduced mortality and complications in surgical patients [3]. The 19 items of the surgical checklist ensure that essential information like patient identity, the type of procedure and its risks (e.g., estimated blood loss), and other patient factors (e.g., allergies) are brought to the team's attention. In addition, equipment issues and anesthetic concerns are checked. This synchronization of essential information is accompanied by an introduction of all team members by name and role in the operating theater. The surgical checklist apparently prevents avoidable human error to a large extent just as the checklist in the B-17 prevented the repetition of the disastrous human error. The surgical checklist additionally aims to improve the communication in the theater team. In theory, better team communication will improve the team response to unexpected events during the course of the procedure.

The training for implementation of the surgical checklist is preferably done in a simulated environment. Importantly, an actual team should train in a simulated environment comparable to the everyday environment. After a theory briefing, the team will observe examples, optionally see film clips, of "How to…" and "How not to do a surgical checklist." The team will then perform a series of checklists interrupted by debriefings. Ideally, two teams train in parallel and observe each other's checklist exercises and participate in the debriefings. This training model is widely used as the surgical checklist currently is implemented across the world. Simulation training is an effective model for training of the surgical checklist since it allows repetitive exercise with interruptive debriefs and the focused attention of the team.

It remains unclear which particular items in the surgical checklist lead to the reduced mortality and complication rate. Interestingly, the positive results were equally significant across continents and cultures. However, the true significance of the results has been questioned since the study design and a possible Hawthorne effect may have biased the result [4].

Beyond reasonable doubt, the surgical checklist obviously meets its demands: preventing avoidable human error. This very purpose of the surgical checklist reflects a true lesson learned from the airline industry as the history of the Boeing prototype and the origin of checklists demonstrates.

In aviation, the application of checklists has expanded from the original purpose, "making sure nothing is overlooked," to a tool for quality control. Checklists are applied in flight operations, technical maintenance and repair, pilot training, and human factors training of both technical and aircraft personnel. Several similarities can be drawn between aviation and surgery, and the application of checklists can potentially expand in surgery. The surgical checklist is comparable to a preflight (sign in and time out) and postflight (sign out) checklist (Table 1.1).

In pilot training, checklists are utilized, e.g., for standardization of operating procedures and for training of reaction patterns to unexpected events. A training checklist for unexpected events (Table 1.2) exercises a safe reaction pattern to those events in the cockpit. Training with this checklist in a safe environment, i.e., in a simulator, prepares the trainee for handling of emergencies in real flight. The reaction pattern is a sequence of actions and/or items to check, predefined by their importance, in order to resolve the situation. Once a technical problem is identified, a specific checklist for the particular system can be gone through.

In principle, a problem or event triggers a response or action algorithm that includes all factors that, in a stressful situation, might be overlooked. Critics claimed

Table 1.1 Checklist for safer surgery as introduced by the World Health Organization

Sign in (before induction of anesthesia)	Patient confirms identity, site of operation, procedure, and consent
	Is the operation site marked?/not applicable
	Anesthesia safety check completed
	Pulse oximeter on patient and functioning
	Patient-specific risk factors:
	• Allergy?
	• Difficult airway/aspiration risk?
	• Risk of >500 mL blood loss (7 mL/kg in children)?
Time out (before skin incision)	All team members introduce themselves by name and role
	Confirmation of patient identification, site of operation, and procedure
	Anticipated critical events:
	• Surgeon reviews: What are the critical or unexpected steps, operative duration, anticipated blood loss?
	• Anesthesia reviews: Are there any patient-specific concerns?
	• Nursing team reviews: Has sterility been confirmed? Are there equipment issues or any concerns?
	Has antibiotic prophylaxis been given?
	Is the essential imaging displayed?
Sign out (before patient leaves operating room)	Verbal confirmation within the team:
	• Name of procedure recorded?
	• Instrument, sponge, and needle count correct?
	• Specimen labeled (if applicable)?
	• Any equipment problems to be addressed?
	Surgeon, anesthesia, and nursing team reviews the key concerns for recovery and postoperative management of the patient

At three timepoints in the operative pathway, essential items are checked. Adjustments are encouraged to fit conditions and requirements of the local institution

with regard to the Boeing prototype crash that the aircraft was "too much airplane to fly for one man." In trauma care, for instance, the initial survey of a critically injured patient requires a rapid evaluation of information and decision-making. In complex cases, the patient might be "too much patient to treat for one surgeon." The Advanced Trauma Life Support (ATLS®) concept resembles an emergency checklist, where the mode of action is predefined by the factors determining outcome [5]. In addition, abbreviations are used in ATLS® (ABCDE) as in the unexpected events checklist in aviation (DECIDE; Table 1.2) to help memorizing the algorithm. After all, the capacity of the human mind is limited in stressful situations as experience in the aviation industry shows. This "task saturation" has been causal to accidents, e.g., when unexpected events or distractions disturb the routine so that some tasks are overlooked, leading to disaster. Quite obviously, surgeons can suffer from task saturation in a routine operation when unexpected events and distractions occur.

Table 1.2 Training checklist for unexpected events

Remain calm, do not rush:
Fly the aircraft, maintain controlled flight—altitude, speed, height
Navigate, avoid terrain, leave bad weather, check fuel
Communicate with your crew and Air Traffic Control; they may be able to help
Review actions already taken
Manage the immediate threat
DECIDE:
D—Detect
Gather all the facts and information about the event—what still works, what does not
E—Estimate
Assess and form an understanding of the situation. Have you seen something similar? Consider possible solutions
C—Choose
Choose the safest practical solution
I—Identify
Identify the actions necessary to carry out the safest option. Have you done this before? What are the expected outcomes?
D—Do
Act, carry out the safest option
E—Evaluate
Evaluate the changes due to the action; reassess the situation, revise the plan if necessary
Review the situation. If it has changed sufficiently, return to the aircraft emergency checklist

Adapted from "Operations Guide to Human Factors in Aviation" issued by the Flight Safety Foundation European Advisory Committee, used with permission [2]

Checklists are also applicable in medical daily routine apart from emergency and unexpected events. Dubose et al. employed a Quality Rounds Checklist (QRC) on a busy intensive care unit (ICU) trauma unit [6]. It contained 16 items focusing on prophylaxis of ICU complications such as ventilator-associated pneumonia (VAP), deep vein thrombosis, and venous catheter infections. After 1 year, the rate of VAPs was reduced by 24%, and the daily use of the QRC had led to a sustained and cost-effective improvement of the complication rate.

In conclusion, checklists have been adapted and utilized in medical practice, e.g., the WHO checklist, for safer surgery and sporadically in other areas. The concept of checklists is yet a familiar concept in medicine as in the ATLS® system. However, the aviation industry has implemented checklists in almost every process from flight operations, maintenance, and human factors training to flight training. Nevertheless, checklists do not prevent all human errors and/or accidents. In fact, relying on checklists can be detrimental. On August 16, 1987, Northwest flight 255 crashed after a "no-flap" takeoff. The following investigation concluded that the pilots were repeatedly distracted while performing the pre-takeoff checklist resulting in the omittance of the correct flap setting for takeoff. Also, the checklist appeared to be

Table 1.3 How to structure the content of a checklist

Chunking	Group items that share a common factor
	Each chunked section should not contain more than nine items
Flow	Items should be listed with a logical progression
Completion call	Each section of the checklist should be completed by a call/answer
Recency	Place the most critical item at the beginning of the list (e.g., patient identity in the WHO checklist)
Redundancy	Repeat critical items to ensure completion (e.g., patient identity in the WHO checklist)
Size	Make the checklist as short as possible but as long as needed

too long and was subsequently divided into several parts in order to facilitate the resumption of the checklist in case of interruption.

Guidelines on the design of an ideal checklist have been issued (Table 1.3). In general, a checklist should be regarded as a dynamic tool of quality control. Its form and content should be audited regularly and amended based on the findings. In fact, the WHO encourages modifications of the safer surgery checklist to meet local demands.

The WHO checklist is one of the available tools for improving patient safety. The checklist principle however, derived from aviation, is applicable to other areas in patient care and training of surgeons.

References

1. Schamel, J. How the pilot's checklist came about. 2009 07.05.2009 [cited 2010 22.02.10]; http://www.atchistory.org/History/checklst.htm]. Accessed 8 Aug 2011.
2. Human Factors, O.S.D., Safety Regulation Group, Civil Aviation Authority UK, Aviation Maintenance Human Factors (JAA JAR145); 2002, Documedia Solutions Ltd, 37 Windsor Street, Cheltenham, Glos., GL52 2DG.
3. Haynes AB, Weiser TG, Berry WR, et al. A surgical safety checklist to reduce morbidity and mortality in a global population. N Engl J Med. 2009;360(5):491–9.
4. Latosinsky S, Thirlby R, Urbach D, et al. CAGS and ACS evidence based reviews in surgery. 32: Use of a surgical safety checklist to reduce morbidity and mortality. Can J Surg. 2010; 53(1):64–6.
5. Jayaraman S, Sethi D. Advanced trauma life support training for hospital staff. Cochrane Database Syst Rev. 2009;(2): CD004173.
6. Dubose J, Teixeira PG, Inaba K, et al. Measurable outcomes of quality improvement using a daily quality rounds checklist: one-year analysis in a trauma intensive care unit with sustained ventilator-associated pneumonia reduction. J Trauma. 2010;69(4):855–60.

Chapter 2
Human Factors, Nontechnical Skills, and Surgical Training

Stig Müller, Waleed Al-Singary, and Hitendra R.H. Patel

Abstract The performance of professionals in the health-care or any other industry is subject to human error. The acknowledgment of human error as ubiquitous and inevitable is the key premise for understanding the importance of human factors. Nontechnical skills (NTS) can improve performance, and attempts have been made to quantify this ambiguous quality. The implementation of NTS into training is possible as experience from flight crew training and aircraft maintenance personnel show. A number of factors that influence human performance negatively have been identified. For instance, stress and fatigue have a negative impact on the performance of surgeons, although this effect to a large extent is neglected among surgeons. Simulation training can facilitate NTS training by integrating elements of, e.g., stress in a simulated environment and thereby prepare surgeons for challenges in patient care and improve surgical training.

S. Müller, M.D., Ph.D. • H.R.H. Patel, MD, PhD (✉)
Department of Urology and Endocrine Surgery,
University Hospital North Norway
Breivika, Tromsø N-9038, Norway
e-mail: hrhpatel@hotmail.com

W. Al-Singary, Dip(Urol), M.Phil., FEB(Urol), FRCS(Urol)
West Sussex Hospital NHS Trust, Sussex Medical Center,
Lyndhurst Road, Worthing, West Sussex, Brighton BN 11 2 DH, UK

Llandough Hospital, Cardiff, UK

Nottingham City Hospital, Nottingham, UK

Benenden Hospital , Kent, UK

Keywords Nontechnical skills • Human factors • Dirty Dozen • Team training Stress

Key Points
- Human error is ubiquitous and inevitable.
- Nontechnical skills are an important adjunct to the performance of professionals.
- The "Dirty Dozen" have adverse effects on human performance.
- Human factors training is an essential part of the training in the aviation industry.
- The importance of human factors in surgery is underrated.
- Stress and fatigue have negative effects on the technical skills of surgeons.
- Nontechnical skills are not automatically acquired by experience.
- Nontechnical skills are trainable in a simulated environment.
- The traditional master-apprentice model in surgical training cannot meet the today's demands of high quality and increasing complexity of procedures.
- New training models that integrate nontechnical skills and modular training are needed.

The cognitive and social skills of experienced professionals have been named "nontechnical skills." These skills are not necessarily acquired by training, yet they augment professional competence. The definition implies that nontechnical skills (NTS) are acquired by experience. However, professional experience does not automatically lead to the acquisition of NTS as experience from the aviation industry and medical training (see below) show. Why are NTS important and how can NTS be trained?

First, one has to realize that human error is ubiquitous and inevitable. In the United States alone, tens of thousands patients die every year from preventable medical errors. The aviation industry has long ago recognized human error as a major cause for hull-loss accidents since approximately 75% of all accidents are caused by human error. This has called for measures to reduce the chance of human error in aviation. Twelve major causes to human error have been identified (Table 2.1). Although derived from aviation, the adverse effect of the "Dirty Dozen" on human performance within health care is obvious. Aviation authorities have initiated

Table 2.1 The "dirty dozen" twelve factors posing a negative influence on human performance

Distraction	Lack of teamwork
Stress	Lack of awareness
Fatigue	Lack of assertiveness
Pressure	Lack of knowledge
Complacency	Lack of communication
Norms	Lack of resources

Table 2.2 Elements of anesthetists' nontechnical skills assessed by the ants-tool [5]

Category	Element
Task management	Planning and preparation
	Prioritization
	Providing and maintaining standards
	Identifying and utilizing resources
Team working	Coordinates activities with team members
	Information exchange
	Use of authority and assertiveness
	Assessment of capabilities of team and self
	Supporting others
Situation awareness	Gathering information
	Understanding and recognition
	Anticipation
Decision making	Identifying
	Balancing risks and selecting options
	Reevaluation

campaigns have tried to raise the awareness of the "Dirty Dozen" in aviation maintenance [1].

At the same time, human factors training has been developed to minimize the impact of human factors that lead to error and accidents. The main objective of human factors training is to reduce error, enhance technical performance, and improve safety. In fact, human factors training has become a requirement for the maintenance industry [2].

While human factors training for maintenance personnel aims to establish a safety-oriented attitude, training for flight crews also needs to focus on personal interactions and teamwork. Over the past decades, Crew Resource Management (CRM) has been developed and has become an integral part of training in aviation [3]. In order to assess NTS and CRM skills, a number of European civil aviation authorities initiated a project in 1996 to identify and develop a taxonomy of pilots' nontechnical skills that would make NTS or CRM skills rateable. The elaborated NOTECHS framework identified four behavioral categories: cooperation, leadership and management skills, situation awareness, and decision making.

These categories have been adapted in the assessment of NTS in operating theaters [4]. The Oxford NOTECHS assessment tool rates the four behavioral categories of NTS, thereby quantifying teamwork. Each category containing more specific elements of behavior is rated on a 4-point scale from "below standard" to "excellent." The reliability and validity has been found sufficient for implementation into clinical practice [4]. A similar system for the assessment of anesthetists' nontechnical skills (ANTS) has also been developed. The categories and elements of behavior have been compiled by a team of anesthetists and psychologists from a series of task analyses based on a literature review, observations, interviews, surveys, and incident analysis. The four main categories of behavior are similar to the NOTECHS and Oxford NOTECHS (Table 2.2).

The ANTS system has been implemented in hospitals in Scotland, and NTS have thus become a focus in clinical practice at the enrolled hospitals. In consequence of the implementation, the positive or negative impact of NTS is reviewed when adverse events are discussed, particularly what behavioral aspect could have influenced or even prevented the adverse event. In these hospitals, the use of ANTS has generated a safety- and quality-orientated attitude. Moreover, ANTS, i.e., education and training in NTS, have become a mandatory part in the training curriculum of junior anesthetists [5].

The ANTS system has been advocated in UK hospitals but the implementation has so far been hesitant, probably due to a lack of enthusiasts as the driving force of the process. Rather than relying on enthusiasts, a sustained implementation of NTS training requires a formal integration into clinical training of specialists, nurses, and others involved in patient care. From the experience in the ANTS system, a training program for anesthetists in NTS terminology and rating tools before implementation has been suggested. Although anesthetic simulators have long been in use, the ANTS system can measure behavioral aspects of anesthetic performance, thus adding a qualitative dimension to the training. Simulation training for laparoscopic surgery has been widely implemented and is effective with regard to the acquisition of technical skills. A variety of models, from simple box-type trainers to virtual reality simulators with haptic feedback, have been validated to improve laparoscopic skills. Also, the transfer of skills acquired in simulators to actual laparoscopic procedures has been documented for, e.g., laparoscopic cholecystectomy [6]. Thus, simulation training improves training and eventually patient outcome. However, this effect is strictly related to technical skills. The importance of technical skills of a surgeon is obvious yet many other factors influence the patient pathway (Fig. 2.1). The acknowledgment of these factors can potentially improve this pathway, especially in unexpected events and when things go wrong.

However, is the focus on NTS beneficial with regard to patient safety or even outcome and furthermore, is NTS training worthwhile?

The rationale for the implementation of NTS training is so far not well founded, although there is evidence that supports the focus on NTS. Stress and fatigue, for instance, are common phenomena and negative factors for professionals. The impact of stress and fatigue is perceived differently among, e.g., medical personnel and flight crews. In a cross-sectional survey of anesthetic nurses and doctors, surgical nurses and doctors, and flight crews, Sexton et al. investigated the professional's attitudes toward error, stress, and teamwork [7]. Medical personnel were more likely to deny the effects of stress and fatigue on their own performance. The perception of teamwork differed among the medical staff. While surgeons generally reported good teamwork with anesthetists, the anesthetic staff did not perceive the same degree of teamwork. Thus, even though NTS training can benefit the different professional groups per se, efforts must be made to include all groups involved in the patient's clinical pathway in a common platform for NTS training. Hierarchy and cultural differences within and across specialties may be the biggest challenges in this process. Flight crew members reported far higher levels of teamwork and advocated flat hierarchies within the team compared to health professionals.

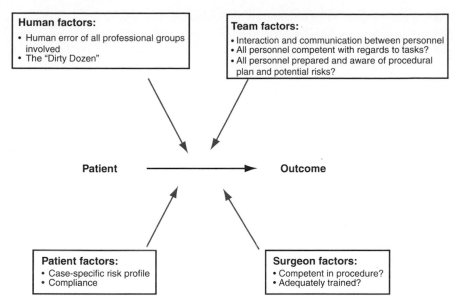

Fig. 2.1 The patient pathway is influenced by different factors

Importantly, flight crews were more aware of the negative effects of stress and fatigue potentially leading to error than medical staff. The acknowledgment of human factors as a cause for error and NTS training has developed a safety- and teamwork-oriented attitude in the airline industry.

Does stress impair performance among medical professionals? In Sexton's survey, intensive-care staff reported poor error management as errors in clinical practice were generally acknowledged but not discussed openly due to various reasons. The acquisition of more staff to deal with the workload was regarded as the most important measure to improve patient safety. A reduction in workload would certainly reduce stress. Surgical staff in large part neglected an impact of fatigue and stress on their performance. However, the negative effect of fatigue on human performance is evident, and the focus on this issue has resulted in working hours directives [8]. Shorter working hours and patient safety requirements create a demand for new and more efficient concepts for surgical training without compromising quality and outcome.

Surgical performance is impaired by stress. Although the objective assessment of surgical skills or performance in a clinical setting is methodologically challenging, several studies in a simulated environment have documented a negative effect of stress on performance [9]. Surgeons regularly experience stress performing surgical procedures dependent on, e.g., level of difficulty or level of training. In laparoscopic surgery in particular, unimpaired dexterity is essential to safely perform a procedure. Thus, the impact of stress in laparoscopic surgery has been investigated in a simulated setting. Stress impairs performance in a simulated setting, and higher levels of stress have an even more adverse effect on performance [10]. However, this relation can be utilized in training. In a study where preclinical medical students performed tasks in a laparoscopic simulator, technical performance, physiologic indicators of stress (blood pressure, heart rate), and pre/post surveys of latent anxiety/stress were observed. The participants performed the tasks with and without a "stressor," a senior faculty member directly observing the performance. The stress levels were highest when the performance was poor under stressor conditions [11]. This study not only shows that stress can be simulated but also that the interactions of stress and performance can be utilized in simulation training.

Is there a need for NTS training, or are NTS acquired with experience? Wetzel et al. conducted a study where 30 surgeons of different seniority performed a carotid endarterectomy in a simulated environment [12]. The procedure was carried out in an uneventful scenario followed by a crisis scenario. Physiologic markers of stress (heart rate, heart variability, salivary cortisol levels) and self-reported/observed psychologic stress levels were recorded. A number of coping strategies were identified, and the technical performance was also assessed. The effect of stress on surgical performance diminished with increasing experience. An experienced surgeon can compensate acute stress with experience without affecting the surgical result. Interestingly, the combination of low experience and low stress was related to poor surgical performance, showing that a certain amount of stress might even be beneficial, at least in inexperienced surgeons. However, coping skills were not associated with experience nor stress, indicating that NTS not automatically are acquired by experience. Coping skills or NTS improve surgical performance and should therefore be integrated in surgical training.

Surgical training is currently challenged by working-hour directives and high-quality standards. The traditional "master-apprentice" model cannot meet the demands of high quality, increasingly complex procedures, and the need for new surgeons. Simulation training is effective and a means to shorten learning curves in laparoscopic surgery. In addition, there are new concepts in training that have been proven effective. In complex laparoscopic surgery, learning curves are often considered to be a measure of how many procedures a trainee has to attend/perform in order to become competent. The sole number of procedures does not, however, reflect the level of difficulty of the case or if the procedure was successful. Thus, a minimum number of procedures do not necessarily lead to competence. In many European countries, this system of a minimum number of different procedures is used in the accreditation of surgeons. Even this quality control appears better than no specified requirements; it is possible to differentiate the factors that determine whether a single procedure is a "rookie" or "expert" case. For instance, in prostate cancer, prostatectomy, prostate size, clinical tumor stage, histological tumor burden, and pelvic comorbidity complicate the procedure and make the procedure more technically challenging.

A preoperative assessment of surgical risk factors also increases the preparedness of the trainee. Breaking down the procedure into steps and subtasks is in this respect beneficial. The trainee can perform single subtasks or steps of the operation that have been assigned different levels of difficulty. This principle is known as modular training. The concept has been validated for, e.g., radical prostatectomy.

Interestingly, the modular approach in training shortens the learning curve significantly without compromising outcome [13, 14].

Another underestimated asset to surgical training is self-observation and assessment. Laparoscopic procedures should in principle be recorded for documentation and the self-assessment of the trainee—preferably together with a mentor—improves training. Such debriefs can be done straight after the procedures or later. The self-observation and assessment shortens the learning curve and is highly motivating for trainees. However, dedicated mentors and time for debriefs must be provided to implement this concept.

The principle of self-assessment is widely used in, e.g., aviation and athletics and has been shown to improve training in a simulated environment. Laparoscopic suturing skills in surgical trainees improve significantly by video self-assessment mirroring the training effect of a larger volume. This training effect is also applicable to single steps or complete procedures.

In conclusion, human factors undoubtedly affect the clinical pathway of a patient, and the "Dirty Dozen" can easily be recognized as negative factors in clinical practice. Training programs should therefore be adapted to include NTS training. Simulation training with adjuncts of NTS training, stress management, and coping strategies will improve the quality of surgical training. NTS training stimulates a quality- and safety-oriented practice. Modular training is a proven concept to shorten learning curves. It can, however, be expanded with preoperative task analysis, case risk assessment, and, importantly, post-procedure video debrief. These different beneficial aspects of training will, when combined, result in a safe and efficient training concept.

References

1. Dupont G. The dirty dozen errors in aviation maintenance. In: Meeting proceedings eleventh Federal Aviation Administration meeting on human factors issues in aircraft maintenance and inspection: human error in aviation maintenance, Washington, D.C.; 1997. p. 45–9.
2. Human Factors, OSD, Safety Regulation Group, Civil Aviation Authority UK, Aviation Maintenance Human Factors (JAA JAR145). 2002, Documedia Solutions Ltd, 37 Windsor Street, Cheltenham, Glos., GL52 2DG.
3. Helmreich RL, Merritt AC, Wilhelm JA. The evolution of Crew Resource Management training in commercial aviation. Int J Aviat Psychol. 1999;9(1):19–32.
4. Mishra A, Catchpole K, McCulloch P. The Oxford NOTECHS System: reliability and validity of a tool for measuring teamwork behavior in the operating theatre. Qual Saf Health Care. 2009;18(2):104–8.
5. Flin R, Patey R, Glavin R, Maran N. Anaesthetists' non-technical skills. Br J Anaesth. 2010;105(1):38–44.
6. Aggarwal R, Crochet P, Dias A, Misra A, Ziprin P, Darzi A. Development of a virtual reality training curriculum for laparoscopic cholecystectomy. Br J Surg. 2009;96:1086–93.
7. Sexton JB, Thomas EJ, Helmreich RL. Error, stress, and teamwork in medicine and aviation: cross sectional surveys. BMJ. 2000;320(7237):745–9.
8. Gaba DM, Howard SK. Patient safety: fatigue among clinicians and the safety of patients. N Engl J Med. 2002;347(16):1249–55.

9. Arora S, Sevdalis N, Nestel D, Woloshynowych M, Drazi A, Kneebone R. The impact of stress on surgical performance: a systematic review of the literature. Surgery. 2010;147(3):318–30, 330 e1–6.
10. Arora S, Sevdalis N, Aggarwal R, Srimanna P, Darzi A, Kneebone R. Stress impairs psychomotor performance in novice laparoscopic surgeons. Surg Endosc. 2010;24(10):2588–93.
11. Andreatta PB, Hillard M, Krain LP. The impact of stress factors in simulation-based laparoscopic training. Surgery. 2010;147(5):631–9.
12. Wetzel CM, Black SA, Hanna GB, Athanasiou T, Kneebone RL, et al. The effects of stress and coping on surgical performance during simulations. Ann Surg. 2010;251(1):171–6.
13. Stolzenburg JU, Rabenalt R, Do M, Horn LC, Liatsikos EN. Modular training for residents with no prior experience with open pelvic surgery in endoscopic extraperitoneal radical prostatectomy. Eur Urol. 2006;49(3):491–8.
14. Ganzer R, Rabenalt R, Truss MC, Papadoukakis S, Do M, et al. Evaluation of complications in endoscopic extraperitoneal radical prostatectomy in a modular training programme: a multicentre experience. World J Urol. 2008;26(6):587–93.

Chapter 3
Current State of Laparoscopic and Robotic Surgery

Jens J. Rassweiler, Marcel Hruza, Thomas Frede, and Salvatore Micali

Abstract Minimally invasive surgical innovation has exploded in recent times. Currently, conventional laparoscopy is most widely adopted as the costs are relatively low. However, robotics and single port surgery are leading a revolution in surgery for wealthy health-care systems. We explore the historical and contemporary areas of this evolution.

Keywords Robotics • Laparoscopy • Surgery • NOTES • LESS • Single port

Key Points
- Laparoscopic surgery is becoming a gold standard across surgical specialities.
- Training in laparoscopy can be difficult and has a significant learning curve.
- Robotic-assisted laparoscopy is expensive but appears easier to learn.
- Single port surgery is novel, offering minimal scars; however, the advantages over conventional laparoscopy are unproven.
- Natural orifice surgery has limitation but has evolved significantly.
- Targeting and image guide surgery are close to adoption.

J.J. Rassweiler, M.D. (✉) • M. Hruza, M.D.
Department of Urology, SLK-Kliniken Heilbronn GmbH,
am Gusuidbrunnen 20-26, Heilbronn 74078, Germany
e-mail: jens.rassweiler@slk-kliniken.de

T. Frede, M.D.
Department of Urology, Helios Kliniken , Heliosreg, Muellheim 79379, Germany

S. Micali, M.D.
Policlinico de Modena, University of Modena & Reggio Emilia,
via del Pozzo, 71, 41100 Modena, Italy

H.R.H. Patel, J.V. Joseph (eds.), *Simulation Training in Laparoscopy and Robotic Surgery*, 15
DOI 10.1007/978-1-4471-2930-1_3, © Springer-Verlag London 2012

Historical Aspects

The Dilemma of the Nineties

Since the early 1990s, laparoscopic surgery has started to become a viable alternative to open surgery for a variety of urological indications (Table 3.1). In contrast to open surgery, where laparoscopic cholecystectomy quickly became the standard approach, there was not such a relatively easy to learn and frequent procedure in urology. Laparoscopic varicocelectomy, even with high success rates (97%), was not widely accepted compared to antegrade or retrograde sclerotherapy. Laparoscopic nephrectomy for benign indications is a rare indication, and in case of non-function hydronephrosis or end-stage stone disease may be really technically challenging. Conclusively, there was the argument that "laparoscopy was a nice procedure looking for an indication."

Nevertheless, pioneers were able to demonstrate the feasibility of laparoscopic ablative as well as reconstructive procedures [1–27]. Since there was a need to overcome the problems of restricted ergonomics particularly concerning endoscopic suturing, several authors focused on the geometrical aspects as well as other ergonomic factors influencing the adequate performance of laparoscopic surgery. Based on this, the first breakthrough was accomplished with the development of a stepwise training for suturing which led to laparoscopic prostatectomy with urethrovesical anastomosis [28–31]. European laparoscopists were able to meet the challenge of

Table 3.1 History of laparoscopy in urology

Indication	Author
Diagnostic of cryptorchidism	Cortesi [1]
Ureterolithotomy	Wickham [2]
Pelvic lymph node dissection	Schüssler [3]
Nephrectomy for oncocytoma	Clayman [4]
Radical nephrectomy for renal cell carcinoma	Coptcoat [5]
Varicocelectomy	Donovan [7]
Nephroureterectomy	Clayman [6]
Pyeloplasty	Kavoussi [8]
Retroperitoneal lymph node dissection	Hulbert [9]
Ileal conduit	Kozminski [10]
Pyelolithotomy	Gaur [12]
Radical cystectomy	Puppo [13]
Living donor nephrectomy	Schulam [14]
Radical prostatectomy	Schuessler [15]
Nephron-sparing excision	Janetschek [16]
Robot-assisted prostatectomy (da Vinci)	Abbou [20]
Radical cystectomy with Mainz-Pouch	Tuerk [22]
Ileal neobladder	Gill [24]
LESS nephrectomy (transumbilical)	Kaouk [26]
NOTES nephrectomy (transvaginal)	Box [27]

this technically difficult procedure, which has now been abandoned by their American colleagues [32–35].

The Diffusion of Laparoscopic Surgery in Urology

With longer follow-up, laparoscopy was able to prove similar oncological results as the open counterpart with respect to radical nephrectomy and nephroureterectomy [36–38]. Based on this, laparoscopic nephrectomy has become the recommended standard in the recent EAU guidelines 2008. The same has been achieved for laparoscopic adrenalectomy; however, this procedure is also performed by general surgeons. In this context, it has to be emphasized that the urological community has not achieved to conduct any prospective randomized multicenter study about the impact of any laparoscopic procedure. This is in contrast to our surgical colleagues who were able to prove the superiority of laparoscopic colectomy [39].

Early in this century, several groups started to perform laparoscopic radical prostatectomy [18, 32, 35]. In the year 2004, about 25% of all radical prostatectomies have been performed laparoscopically in Germany [40, 41]. However, there is still the debate about the superiority of this procedure over the standard retropubic open approach [42–44]. There is consensus that still the surgeon represents the most important factor of success [44]. Other laparoscopic reconstructive procedures, such as pyeloplasty or sacrocolpopexy, gained interest and some centers receive referrals particularly for these indications [45–47].

The Revolution of Robotic Surgery

This time, everything started in Europe with the first cases of robotic-assisted laparoscopic radical prostatectomies using the da Vinci device at the beginning of this century [19, 20, 48, 49] (Table 3.1). However, the procedure did not gain significant attraction mainly due to the enormous costs. Moreover, the patients did not demand the procedure. In the United States, the story of success of the da Vinci prostatectomy happened completely unexpected. The significantly improved ergonomics of the device with the surgeon sitting at the console using 3D vision and instruments with 7 degrees of freedom alleviated the introduction of laparoscopic surgery even for surgeons without any laparoscopic experience [50].

The most important factor represented the marketing strategy in the United States, where reimbursement was not a significant problem and "the robot" proved to be extremely attractive for the patient. Based on this, in 2009 almost 80% of all radical prostatectomies have been performed laparoscopically using the da Vinci device. Additionally, the robot is used increasingly for partial nephrectomies and pyeloplasties [51]. Again, there is not a single randomized study comparing open surgery to the robotic-assisted laparoscopy.

At the beginning, some specific difficulties of the da Vinci system have been encountered particularly for surgeons with laparoscopic experience [49].

Interpretation of Magnified Anatomy

The first problem for a laparoscopic surgeon represents the interpretation of the respective anatomical structures (i.e., the dorsal vein complex, bladder neck, vas deferens) seen under stereoscopic vision with a tenfold magnification. It proved to be difficult to adjust the new image to the known two-dimensional picture one has been used to over the last decade. The same applies to identify small vessels.

Lack of Tactile Feedback

The lack of haptic sense aggravates the dissection technique in this novel situation. Even if "standard" laparoscopy does only provide a minimal amount of tactile sensation, the effect of training and experience finally enabled the surgeon to have a certain haptic sensation, i.e., to assess the shape of the prostate, the severity of adhesions, and the strength of a suture or knot. The da Vinci system, actually, does not provide any tactile feedback. Nevertheless, the surgeon is able to compensate the missing tactile feedback by the improved stereoscopic vision (i.e., observing the deformation of tissue and the increasing tension on the suture). With increasing experience, one is able to estimate the applied strength on the suture when performing a knot. Nevertheless, working remotely without tactile feedback requires new surgical skills, solely based on visual inputs. This of course increases the mental stress during surgery.

Coordinated Interaction Between Surgeon and Assistants

The complexity of the operation itself requires proper assistance and instrumentation. In contrast to a laparoscopic nephrectomy or adrenalectomy, a laparoscopic radical prostatectomy cannot be performed as solo surgery. There is a need of retraction of the gland or adjacent structures. For vascular control, clips have to be placed, and sometimes suction is required to clear the operating field. All this has to be carried out by the assistant working under a deteriorated ergonomic situation.

Ergonomic Advantages of the da Vinci System

In robotic surgery, the working ergonomy for the surgeon is optimized due to the seated position, the clutch function, the tremor filter, and the in-line 3D vision. It is important to note that the sitting position alone does not improve the performance as shown by Berguer and Smith with the ZEUS device lacking the 7-DOF [52]. Moreover, at the da Vinci robot, the surgeon himself controls the camera. On the other hand, there is no tactile feedback, and the surgeon is very much dependent on optimal assistance (i.e., placement of clips). The working ergonomy for certain steps of the procedure can be even worse than during standard laparoscopy because of the robotic arms interfering with the manipulations of the assistant. The introduction of the fourth arm has improved this with respect to proper tissue retraction and exposure of the working field, but the situation for the assistant remains unchanged. Moreover, the mental stress on the surgeon at the console controlling five foot pedals and two arm handles (plus the fourth arm) should not be underestimated.

Newest Technological Developments

Recently, our attention has been focused on a modification of laparoscopy, the transition from multiple to single port access: Laparo-Endoscopic Single-Site Surgery (LESS). Reworked from an old technique, pioneered by gynecologists in the 1960s [53], they used an operative laparoscope, comparable to a rigid nephroscope, for tubal ligation. LESS has become attractive for multiple procedures [26]. In addition, abdominal targets have been approached in a transluminal way via natural orifices (i.e., mouth, vagina, anus, and urethra) leaving the patient without any scar [54]. Recently, NOTES (natural orifice transluminal endoscopic surgery) has been also tested for urological indications [25, 27].

Laparo-Endoscopic Single Port Surgery (LESS)

LESS is the standard term designated to avoid confusion and acronyms. It represents any minimally invasive intra-abdominal surgical procedure performed through a single incision/location, utilizing conventional laparoscopic or newly emerging instruments. Any procedures performed with an additional transperitoneal port should be referred to as hybrid LESS.

Raman et al. reported a successful experiment with a LESS nephrectomy on a porcine model and in human subjects [55]. Other small series show similar outcomes: live donor nephrectomy, renal cryotherapy, varicocelectomy, simple and even radical prostatectomy [26, 56–58]. About 100 abstracts describing LESS case report (ileal conduit, sacrocolpopexy, partial cystectomy) were presented at the WCE 2008 (Table 3.2) [20, 21]. At the WCE 2009, there were more series and comparative studies, revealing excellent cosmetics results and less pain over standard laparoscopy (Table 3.3) [20, 21].

The LESS technique involves main access ports via a single incision (2–3 cm). Articulated and pre-bent instruments allow for intracorporeal triangulation,

Table 3.2 Summary of less results at the World Congress on Endourology and SWL 2008 and 2009

Authors	Year	Procedures	Pts	LESS technique	Conclusions
White W. et al. MP18–16[a]	2008	Renal (29) and pelvic (22) surgery 8 retroperitoneal access	51[c]		"Its superiority as compared to traditional laparoscopy is currently speculative"
Desai M. et al. MP18–12[a]	2008	Transvesical prostate enucleation	15	R-Port ultrasonic shears	"Early experience appears encouraging"
Schwartz M. et al. VP8–02[b]	2009	Pyeloplasty (41)—7 hybrid	41		".... particularly advantageous in young patients more concerned with cosmesis"
Desai M et al. VP8–01[b]	2009	Renal (51), prostate (32), and others (11)	100[d]	R-Port + 2 mm grasper	"Improvement in instrumentation and technology is likely to expand the role of LESS"

[a]Abstracts presented at the 26th WCE & SWL 2008
[b]Abstracts presented at the 27th WCE & SWL 2009
[c]7 Renal cryoablations, 6 partial, 4 simple, 3 radical nephrectomies, 1 retroperitoneal mass ablation, 1 renal biopsy, 2 cyst ablation, 2 pyeloplasty, 3 nephroureterectomies, 3 varicocelectomies, 5 prostatectomy, 3 cystectomy, 1 ureteral reimplantation, 10 colposacropexy
[d]14 simple, 3 radical, 17 donor nephrectomies, 17 pyeloplasty, 32 simple

Table 3.3 Comparative study LESS versus laparoscopy presented at World Congress on Endourology 2008 and 2009

Nephrectomy 22 LESS vs. 11 Lap	33	Three adjacent 5 mm trocars	"LESS may offer a subjective cosmetic advantage"
Live donor nephrectomy 9 LESS vs. 9 Lap	18	R-Port	"LESS offers quicker convalescence and longer warm ischemia time"
Pyeloplasty 8 LESS vs. 8 Lap	16	R-Port+2 mm grasper	"LESS offers better convalescence and cosmetic benefits"
Partial nephrectomy 15 LESS vs. 15 Lap	30	n.a.Hybrid	"LESS offers equivalent comparative outcomes, significant less pain, and superior cosmesis"
Renal cyst marsupialization 15 LESS vs. 14 Lap	29	Homemade port from surgical glove	"LESS could be considered as primary treatment option"

despite adjacent position of trocars. Bent instruments are reusable and thus more cost-effective than articulated devices. However, the restriction on the degrees of freedom might result in a steeper learning curve than with articulating instruments. In comparison to the conventional laparoscopy, there are three main problems:

Triangulation: Instrument triangulation allows proper tissue retraction. Parallel placement of several instruments makes triangulation more difficult. However, using at least one flexible or curved instrument may offset the shafts adequately and accomplish a satisfactory degree of triangulation.

Retraction: The lack of additional assistant trocars limits correct exposition of structures. These can be achieved with intra-abdominal sutures affixed to the parietal peritoneum or transcutaneous sutures grasped and manipulated extracorporeally.

Instrument crowding: The parallel placement and proximity of instruments may result in their crowding. Clashing of instruments could be avoided by using bent, articulated, and different length instruments (i.e., obese and pediatric equipment). Moreover, recently developed laparoscopes (i.e., Endo-Eye, Olympus, Hamburg, Germany) offer a streamlined profile compared to the standard laparoscopic light cable entering the lens at 90°, where interaction with adjacent instruments is severely limited.

Transvesical LESS eliminates the contact with the peritoneal cavity and provides a direct inline exposition of the prostate obviating the need for mobilizing the bladder and developing the Retzius space. Desai et al. reported simple prostatectomy (three patients) and even robotic LESS radical prostatectomies [58].

Natural Orifice Transluminal Endoscopic Surgery (NOTES)

NOTES is defined as a surgical procedure that utilizes one or more natural orifices (i.e., mouth, anus, vagina, urethra), with the intention to puncture hollow viscera (i.e., bladder, vagina, colon, stomach), in order to enter the abdomen. Hybrid NOTES should be considered when additional instruments are placed transabdominally to assist the NOTES procedure [10].

Breda et al. for the first time described a vaginal extraction of a kidney following laparoscopic nephrectomy [59]. Gettman ct al. reported a transvaginal hybrid NOTES nephrectomy in the porcine model [25]. NOTES developed significantly following the report of transgastric liver biopsy and cholecystectomy by Kalloo et al. in the animal model [60]. Since then, laboratory and clinical reports included cholecystectomy, tubal ligation, splenectomy, and appendectomy. Selection of best portal access needs to consider many factors: ease of access and closure, risk of infection, and relationship to the target anatomy (Table 3.4).

Transgastric: After advancing the endoscope into the stomach, the anterior abdominal wall is trans-illuminated and punctured with a needle or a needle-knife. A guide wire is advanced into the peritoneal cavity, a sphinctertome is inserted, and a gastric incision performed (comparable to PEG). Gastrotomy closure is accomplished either with endoclips or suturing devices [54]. Kalloo et al. evaluated the gastrointestinal tract to perform successful peritoneoscopy, liver biopsy, and gastric closure with clips in six pigs. At sacrifice, peritoneal cultures were negative [60]. A recent review described the first appendectomy on a human using the same technique.

Table 3.4 Different approaches to NOTES

Translumenal approach	Comments
Transgastric	(+) Well-known and safe procedure used to create PEG
	(−) Barriers still exist: standardization of gastrotomy site, endoscopic retroflection for upper abdominal procedures, spatial orientation, and optimal closure technique
Transvaginal	(+) Readily secure closure offered by standard surgical technique
	(−) Gynecologists claim postoperative infection, visceral lesions, infertility, and adhesions as conceivable complications. Other long-term potential problems could be dyspareunia, infertility, and the spread of preexisting endometriosis [48]
Transcolonic	(+) Well tolerated and offers easy access to multiple targets, even retroperitoneum and easy visualization of upper abdominal organs. Colon compliance could tolerate larger instrument and specimen retrieval
	(−) An incomplete closure of the colostomy site and subsequent peritonitis will be catastrophic
Transvesical	(+) Allows for a direct visualization of all intra-abdominal structures. The urinary tract is normally sterile and the risk of infection and intraperitoneal or retroperitoneal contamination should be less. Cystostomy sites are known to heal spontaneously by catheter drainage
	(−) Diameter of urethra can limit instruments introduction

Transvaginal: The posterior vaginal fornix is opened using a special trocar and the pouch of Douglas is reached, saline solution is injected, and a 2.7-mm endoscope is then introduced.

Gettman et al. described the first experimental transvaginal application of NOTES: a transvaginal nephrectomy on a porcine model [25]. Nowadays, the vagina is the most frequently used access route for clinical NOTES, but also criticized, because this may cause problems during intercourse.

Transcolonic: The site of access is 15–20 cm from the anus. A specially designed guide tube (ISSA) is inserted via the colon into the abdominal cavity after intraperitoneal instillation of a decontamination solution [61]. The technique of closure includes endoscopic clips and prototype stapling devices. Pai et al. performed in a porcine survival model transcolonic cholecystectomy. All animals survived postoperatively without signs of infection; however, on necropsy animals evidenced intraperitoneal adhesion and microabscesses [62]. Other applications included distal pancreatectomy and ventral hernia repair [61].

Transvesical: A flexible injection needle is advanced through the working channel of a cystoscope or ureteroscope to perforate the bladder dome. A balloon dilator is then passed over a guide wire to enlarge the cystostomy tract. Lima et al. [63] performed peritoneum cavity inspection, liver biopsy, and division of the falciform ligament in animal model. Bladder catheter was left 4 days and on necropsy after 15 days all cystostomies healed. The same authors performed in a porcine model a combined transvesical/transgastric hybrid NOTES cholecystectomy and a transvesical thoracoscopy access [64].

Limitation of Notes in Urology

At the WCE 2008 and 2009, a total of five abstracts described feasibility of trans-vaginal nephrectomy in human [27]. A recent study summarized the clinical application of NOTES analyzing 16 publications and highlighting great difficulties: 46 of 49 procedures required conversion to hybrid NOTES [65]. Lima et al. described a third-generation nephrectomy combining transgastric and transvesical NOTES. They concluded that this approach is technically feasible; however, there is no reliable method for removing the specimen [64].

This technique still lacks available instrumentation. Most of the reported surgical experience concludes that there is no technological advancement on this topic. The development of novel suturing and articulated instruments, flexible bipolar forceps, clips and staplers as well as the advent of manual mechanical manipulators for flexible accessories is outlined in Table 3.5. Moreover, the risk of the access-induced

Table 3.5 Available tools to perform NOTES in urology

Categories of instruments	Tools	Description/comment
Peritoneoscopes	Conventional gastroscope	(−) Inadequate illumination
		Floppy nature: Limited control of the tip
		Flexible instruments are ineffective for retraction and grasping tissue
		Not suitable for CO_2 insufflation (leakage and impossible pressure control)
	R-Scope (Olympus America, Center Valley, PA, USA)	Two elevators at the tip allow flexible instrument to be moved
NOTES platforms	Cobra (USGI Medical, San Clemente, CA, USA)	Two arms allow triangulation and rigidization
	USGI TransPort™ (USGI Medical, San Clemente, CA, USA)	18 mm Ø; 4 channels (7, 6, 4, and 4 mm)
		ShapeLock technology allows to be locked into desired shape, even when rigid distal section can be steered
Dissections	Spray Dissector (Ethicon Endo-Surgery, Cincinnati, Ohio)	Tip buried inside ceramic tip
Hemostasis	Flexible bipolar hemostasis forceps (Ethicon Endo-Surgery, Cincinnati, Ohio, USA)	Coagulation intraperitoneal vessel up to 4 mm in diameter
Clips	Triclips (Cook Endoscopy, Winston-Salem, NC, USA)	
	Resolution Clips (Boston Scientific, Natick, MA, USA)	
	Rotating clips (Olympus)	
Closure	T-tag	
	G-Prox tissue suturing system	

injury (i.e., peritonitis) has to be balanced with the complications of a standard laparoscopic or LESS procedure.

Future Directions

It has to be emphasized that the technical principle of laparoscopy and retroperitoneoscopy has proven to be safe and effective. Based on this, the technique has found acceptance in recent guidelines (Table 3.6).

New developments are only related to the modification of these minimally invasive techniques, be it by the assistance of a robot or using a single port. To further reduce the invasiveness of laparoscopy, surgeons have proposed limiting the number of abdominal incision (LESS) or eliminating them completely (NOTES). Best aesthetic results and less postoperative pain offered by LESS are clearly visible. Anyway only a long-term follow-up will assess functional and oncological results versus traditional laparoscopy. Moreover, the future will show how much a scar really matters. This may be different in certain parts of the world. In Brazil, LESS and NOTES have become very demanded by female patients. NOTES perfectly fit role of scar-free surgery and multiple routes of access have been shown safe and effective. However, only few studies on human have been accomplished, and many authors agree that the lack of applied instrument did avoid the determination of the real role of NOTES in clinical practice. Combination of robotics and augmented reality could be the next step for NOTES evolutions [66–68].

There is a need to improve the ergonomics of traditional laparoscopic surgery. The design of the da Vinci robot offers a variety of ergonomic advantages compared to pure laparoscopy. However, there are also some disadvantages, such as the lack of tactile feedback and restricted ergonomics for the assistant. The impact of these advantages depends also on the type of the procedure. There will be new robots on the market, providing even haptic sense, such as the project of the German Aerospace Research Centre on the construction of modular robot system for minimally invasive surgery (MiroSurge). In contrast to the da Vinci system, the robotic arms are controlled by micromotors allowing easy adjustment of the arms at the OR table (Fig. 3.1a).

Table 3.6 Differential indications for laparoscopic techniques in the year 2010

Indication	Laparoscopy	Robotic (da Vinci)	LESS
Adrenalectomy	First line	Not applied	Optional
Radical nephrectomy	First line	Not applied	Optional
Simple nephrectomy	First line	Not applied	Optional
Living donor nephrectomy	First line/optional	Not applied	Experimental
Partial nephrectomy	Optional	Optional	Experimental
Radical prostatectomy	Optional	First line/optional	Experimental
Radical cystectomy	Optional	Optional	Not applied
Pyeloplasty	First line	Optional	Optional
Sacrocolpopexy	Optional	Optional	Experimental

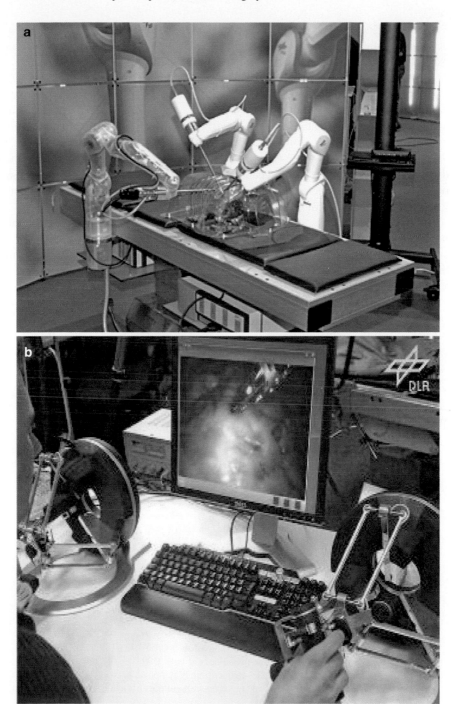

Fig. 3.1 New robotic device MiroSurge from the project of the German Aerospace Research Centre. (**a**) The robotic arms are controlled by micromotors, allowing easy adjustment of the arms at the operating room table. (**b**) The surgeon sits at a console using an autostereoscopic 3D monitor and two specially designed handles with integrated force feedback

The surgeon sits at a console using an autostereoscopic 3D monitor and two specially designed handles with integrated force feedback. The device has been a construction parallel to remote controlled robots used in space (Fig. 3.1b).

On the other hand, efforts should be undertaken by all manufacturers involved in the design of the operating theater to focus on the improvement of ergonomics according to the existing guidelines. This concerns the design of armamentarium and instruments, but also the OR table, platforms, OR chairs, arrangement of lines and cables. Some of this will include the perfection of already existing 7-DOF-devices for laparoscopy (i.e., equipped with miniaturized motors) [69, 70], the design of camera holders (i.e., compared to AESOP), and the improvement of LESS ports, providing completely steerable working channels for the flexible instruments to avoid any crossing of the instruments.

With all these new technical improvements, traditional laparoscopy will become much easier to perform. However, the success of the robot will not be stopped by any means. Similarly to the history of shock wave lithotripsy, cost arguments will become less important in the future. Every surgeon who successfully passed the learning curve of the da Vinci device never went back to open surgery. Of course experienced laparoscopists will still select cases for all three options (i.e., laparoscopy, LESS, robotic surgery; Table 3.6). On the other hand, the future of NOTES (i.e., with a transvaginal or transvesical access) still remains uncertain. It will be difficult to understand why a transvaginal access should be superior to a transumbilical port followed by a meticulous umbilicoplasty.

References

1. Cortesi N, Ferrari P, Zambarda E, Manetti A, Baldini A, Morano FP. Diagnosis of bilateral abdominal cryptorchidism by laparoscopy. Endoscopy. 1976;8:33–7.
2. Wickham JEA. The surgical treatment of renal lithiasis. In: Wickham JEA, editor. Urinary calculus disease. New York: Churchill Livingstone; 1979. p. 145–98.
3. Schüssler WW, Vancaillie TG, Reich H, Griffith DP. Transperitoneal endosurgical lymphadenectomy in patients with localized prostrate cancer. J Urol. 1991;145:988–91.
4. Clayman RV, Kavoussi LR, Soper NJ, Dierks SM, Meretyk S, Darcy MD, Roemer FD, Pingleton ED, Thomson PG, Long SR. Laparoscopic nephrectomy: initial case report. J Urol. 1991;146:278–82.
5. Coptcoat MJ, Rassweiler J, Wickham JEA, Joyce A, Popert R. Laparoscopic nephrectomy for renal cell carcinoma. In: Proceedings of the third international congress for minimal invasive therapy, Boston, 10–12 Nov 1991 (abstract No. D-66).
6. Clayman RV, Kavoussi LR, Figenshau RS, Chandhoke P, Albala DM. Laparoscopic nephroureterectomy: initial clinical case report. J Laparoendocopic Surg. 1991;1:343–9.
7. Donovan JF, Winfield HN. Laparoscopic varix ligation. J Urol. 1992;147:77–81.
8. Kavoussi LR, Peters CA. Laparoscopic pyeloplasty. J Urol. 1993;150:1891–4.
9. Hulbert JC, Fraley EE. Laparoscopic retroperitoneal lymphadenectomy: new approach to pathologic staging of clinical stage I germ cell tumors of the testis. J Endourol. 1992;6:123–5.
10. Kozminski M, Partamian KO. Case report of laparoscopic ileal loop conduit. J Endourol. 1992;6:147–50.

11. Parra RO, Andrus CH, Jones JP, Boullier JA. Laparoscopic cystectomy: initial report on a new treatment for the retained bladder. J Urol. 1992;148:1140–4.
12. Gaur DD, Agarwal DK, Purohit KC, Darshane AS. Retroperitoneal laparoscopic pyelolithotomy. J Urol. 1994;151:927–9.
13. Puppo P, Perachino M, Ricciotti G, Bozzo W, Gallucci M, Carmignani G. Laparoscopically assisted transvaginal radical cystectomy. Eur Urol. 1995;27:80–4.
14. Schulam PG, Kavoussi LR, Cheriff AD, Averch TD, Montgomery R, Moore RG, Ratner LE. Laparoscopic live donor nephrectomy: the initial 3 cases. J Urol. 1996;155:1857–9.
15. Schuessler W, Schulam P, Clayman R, Kavoussi L. Laparoscopic radical prostatectomy: initial short-term experience. Urology. 1997;50:854–7.
16. Janetschek G, Daffner P, Peschel R, et al. Laparoscopic nephron sparing surgery for small renal cell carcinoma. J Urol. 1998;159:1152–5.
17. Guillonneau B, Vallancien G. Laparoscopic radical prostatectomy: the Montsouris experience. J Urol. 2000;163:418–22.
18. Rassweiler J, Sentker L, Seemann O, Hatzinger M, Rumpelt J. Laparoscopic radical prostatectomy with the Heilbronn technique: an analysis of the first 180 cases. J Urol. 2001;160:201–8.
19. Binder J, Kramer W. Robotically assisted laparoscopic radical prostatectomy. BJU Int. 2001;87:408–10.
20. Abbou CC, Hoznek A, Salomon L, Olsson LE, Lobontiu A, Saint F, Cicco A, Antiphon P, Chopin D. Laparoscopic radical prostatectomy with a remote controlled robot. J Urol. 2001;165:1964–6.
21. Denewer A, Kotb S, Hussein O, El-Maadawy M. Laparoscopic assisted cystectomy and lymphadenectomy for bladder cancer: initial experience. World J Surg. 1999;23:608.
22. Türk I, Deger S, Winkelmann B, Schönberger B, Loening SA. Laparoscopic radical cystectomy with continent urinary diversion (rectal sigmoid pouch) performed completely intracorporeally: the initial 5 cases. J Urol. 2001;165:1863–966.
23. Gaboardi F, Simonate A, Galli S, Lissiani A, Gregori A, Bozzola A. Minimally invasive laparoscopic neobladder. J Urol. 2002;168:1080–3.
24. Gill IS, Kaouk JH, Meraney AM, Desai MM, Ulchaker JC, Klein EA, Savage SJ, Sung GT. Laparoscopic radical cystectomy and continent orthotopic ileal neobladder performed completely intracorporeally: the initial experience. J Urol. 2002;168:13–8.
25. Gettman MT, Lotan Y, Napper CA, et al. Transvaginal laparoscopic nephrectomy: development and feasibility in the porcine model. Urology. 2002;59:446–50.
26. Kaouk JH, Haber GP, Goel RK, Desai M, Aron M, Rackley RR, Moore C, Gill IS. Single-port laparoscopic surgery in urlogy: initial experience. Urology. 2008;71:3–6.
27. Box GN, Lee HJ, Santos RJS, et al. Rapid communication. Robot-Assisted NOTES Nephrectomy: initial report. J Endourol. 2008;22(3):503–5.
28. Frede T, Stock C, Renner C, Budair Z, Abdel-Salam Y, Rassweiler J. Geometry of laparoscopic suturing and knotting techniques. J Endourol. 1999;13:191–8.
29. Frede T, Stock C, Rassweiler JJ, Alken P. Retroperitoneoscopic and laparoscopic suturing: tips and strategies for improving efficiency. J Endourol. 2000;14:905–13.
30. Hemal AK, Srinivas M, Charles AR. Ergonomic problems associated with laparoscopy. J Endourol. 2001;15:499–503.
31. Berguer R. Ergonomics and laparoscopic surgery. Laparoscopy Today. 2005;4:8–11.
32. De la Rosette JJMCH, Abbou CC, Rassweiler J, Pilar LM, Schulman CC. Laparoscopic radical prostatectomy: a European virus with global potential. Arch Esp Urol. 2002;55:603–9.
33. Rassweiler J, Seemann O, Schulze M, Teber D, Hatzinger M, Frede T. Laparoscopic versus open radical prostatectomy: a comparative study at a single institution. J Urol. 2003;169:1689–93.
34. Rassweiler J, Frede T, Guillonneau B. Advanced laparoscopy. Eur Urol. 2002;42:1 (Curric Urol 1–12).
35. Rassweiler J, Hruza M, Teber D, Su L-M. Laparoscopic and robotic assisted radical prostatectomy – critical analysis of the results. Eur Urol. 2006;49:612–24.

36. Dunn MD, Portis AJ, Shalhav AL, Elbahnasy AM, Heidorn C, McDougall EM, Clayman RV. Laparoscopic versus open radical nephrectomy: a 9-year experience. J Urol. 2000;164:1153–9.
37. El Fetouh HA, Rassweiler JJ, Schulze M, Salomon L, Allan J, Ramakumar S, Jarrett T, Abbou CC, Tolley DA, Kavoussi LR, Gill IS. Laparoscopic radical nephroureterectomy: results of an international multicenter study. Eur Urol. 2002;42:447–52.
38. Rassweiler JJ, Schulze MM, Marrero R, Frede T, Palou Redorta J, Bassi P. Laparoscopic nephroureterectomy for upper urinary tract transitional cell carcinoma: is it better than open surgery? Eur Urol. 2004;46:690–7.
39. Clinical outcomes of surgical therapy study group. A comparison of laparoscopically assisted and opne colectomy for colon cancer. N Engl J Med. 2004;350:2050–9.
40. Vögeli TA, Burchardt M, Fornara P, Rassweiler J, Sulser T. Laparoscopic Working Group of the German Urological Association: current laparoscopic practice patterns in urology: results of a survey among urologists in Germany and Switzerland. Eur Urol. 2002;42:441–6.
41. Rassweiler J, Stolzenburg J, Sulser T, Deger S, Zumbé J, Hofmockel G, John H, Janetschek G, Fehr J-L, Hatzinger M, Probst M, Rothenberger H, Poulakis V, Truss M, Popken G, Westphal J, Alles U, Fornara P. Laparoscopic radical prostatectomy – the experience of the German Laparoscopic Working Group. Eur Urol. 2006;49:113–9.
42. Rassweiler J, Schulze M, Teber D, Marrero R, Seemann O, Rumpelt J, Frede T. Laparoscopic radical prostatectomy with the Heilbronn technique: oncological results in the first 500 patients. J Urol. 2005;173:761–4.
43. Guazzoni G, Cestari A, Naspro R, Riva M, Centernero A, Zanoni M, Rigatti L, Rigatti P. Intra- and peri-operative outcomes comparing radical retropubic and laparoscopic radical prostatectomy: Results from a prospective, randomized, single-surgeon study. Eur Urol. 2006;50:98–104.
44. Ficarra V, Novara G, Artibani W, et al. Retropubic, laparoscopic, and robot-assisted radical prostatectomy: a systematic review and cumulative analysis of comparative studies. Eur Urol. 2009;55(5):1037–63.
45. Antiphon P, Elard S, Benyoussef A, Fofana M, Yiou R, Gettman M, Hoznek A, Vordos D, Chopin DK, Abbou CC. Laparoscopic promontory sacral colpopexy: is the posterior, recto-vaginal mesh mandatory? Eur Urol. 2004;45:655–61.
46. Rozet F, Mandron E, Arroyo C, Andrews H, Cathelineau X, Mombet A, Cathala N, Vallancien G. Laparoscopic sacral colpopexy approach for genito-urinary prolapse: experience with 363 cases. Eur Urol. 2005;47:230–6.
47. Rassweiler JJ, Subotic S, Feist-Schwenk M, Sugiono M, Schulze M, Teber D, Frede T. Minimally invasive treatment of ureteropelvic junction obstruction: long-term experience with an algorhythm for laser endopyelotomy and laparoscopic retroperitoneal pyeloplasty. J Urol. 2007;177:1000–5.
48. Rassweiler J, Frede T, Seemann O, Stock C, Sentker L. Telesurgical laparoscopic radical prostatectomy – intial experience. Eur Urol. 2001;40:75–83.
49. Rassweiler J, Binder J, Frede T. Robotic and telesurgery: will they change our future? Curr Opin Urol. 2001;11:309–20.
50. Hemal AK, Menon M. Robotics in urology. Curr Opin Urol. 2004;14:89–93.
51. Thield DD, Winfield HD. Robotics in urology: past, present and future. J Endourol. 2008;2(4):825–30.
52. Berguer R, Smith W. An ergonomic comparison of robotic and laparoscopic technique: the influence of surgeon experience and task complexitiy. J Surg Res. 2006;134:87–92.
53. Wheeless CR. A rapid, inexpensive and effective method of surgical sterilization by laparoscopy. J Reprod Med. 1969;5:255–7.
54. Swain P. Nephrectomy and Natural Orifice Translumenal Endosurgery (NOTES): transvaginal, transgastric, transrectal, and transvescical approaches. J Endourol. 2008;22(4):811–7.
55. Raman JD, Bagrodia A, Cadeddu JA. Single-incision, umbilical laparoscopic versus conventional laparoscopic nephrectomy: a comparison of peri-operative outcomes and short-term measures of convalescence. Eur Urol. 2009;55(5):1198–204.

56. Desai MM, Aron M, Canes D, et al. Single-port transvesical simple prostatectomy: initial clinical report. Urology. 2008;72(2):960–5.
57. Kaouk JH, Goel RK, Haber G, et al. Single-port laparoscopic radical prostatectomy. Urology. 2008;72(6):1191–3.
58. Desai MM, Aron M, Canes D, et al. Single-port transvesical simple prostatectomy: initial clinical report. J Urol. 2008;72(5):960–5.
59. Breda G, Silvestre P, Giunta A, et al. Laparoscopic nephrectomy with vaginal delivery of the intact kidney. Eur Urol. 1993;24:116–7.
60. Kalloo AN, Singh VK, Jagannath SB, et al. Fexible transgastric peritoneoscopy: a novel approach to diagnostic and therapeutic interventions in the peritoneal cavity. Gastrointest Endosc. 2004;60:114–7.
61. Shin EJ, Kalloo AN. Transcolonic NOTES: current experience and potential implications for urologic applications. J Endourol. 2009;23(5):743–6.
62. Pai RD, Fong DG, Bundga ME, Odze RD, Rattner DW, Thompson CC. Transcolonic endoscopic cholecystectomy: a NOTES survival study in a porcine model. Gastrointest Endosc. 2006;64:428–34.
63. Lima E, Rolanda C, Pego JM, et al. Transvesical endoscopic peritoneoscopy: a novel 5 mm port for intra-abdominal scarless surgery. J Urol. 2006;176:802–5.
64. Lima E, Rolanda C, Pego JM, et al. Third-generation nephrectomy by natural orifice transluminal endoscopic surgery. J Urol. 2007;178:2648–54.
65. Xavier K, Gupta M, Landman J. Transgrastric NOTES: current experience and potential implications for urological applications. J Endourol. 2009;23(5):737–41.
66. Rassweiler J, Baumhauer M, Weickert U, Meinzer HP, Teber D, Su LM, Patel VR. The role of imaging and navigation for natural orifice translumenal endoscopic surgery. J Endourol. 2009;23:793–802.
67. Teber D, Baumhauer M, Guven EO, Rassweiler J. Robotic and imaging in urological surgery. Curr Opin Urol. 2009;19:108–13.
68. Haber GP, Crouzet S, Kamoi K, Berger A, Aron M, Goel R, Canes D, Desai M, Gill AI, Kaouk JH. Robotic NOTES (Natural Orifice Transluminal Endoscopic Surgery) in reconstructive urology: initial laboratory experience. Urology. 2008;71(6):996 1000.
69. Frede T, Hammady A, Klein J, Teber D, Inaki N, Waseda M, Buess G, Rassweiler J. The Radius Surgical System – a new device for complex minimally invasive procedures in urology? Eur Urol. 2007;51:1015–22.
70. Kenngott HG, Müller-Stich BP, Reiter MA, Rassweiler J, Gutt CN. Robotic suturing: technique and benefit of advanced laparoscopic surgery. Minim Invasive Ther Allied Technol. 2008;17:160–7.

Chapter 4
Simulation and Training in Minimally Invasive Surgery

Sonal Arora, Shabnam Undre, and Roger Kneebone

Abstract Changes to the delivery of surgical services, shortened training times, and an increasing awareness of patient safety have had a profound effect on surgical training. Urology is a technology-driven specialty, in which the impact of such changes is potentially critical. Surgical training has traditionally relied upon direct patient care, but the tide is now turning. As laparoscopy and other minimally invasive urological techniques are introduced, there is an opportunity to explore alternative teaching and training strategies. Simulation is becoming increasingly embraced in urology training programs. This chapter provides an overview of the background of simulation for minimally invasive surgery and explores its potential to provide technical and nontechnical skills training for urologists.

Keywords Surgery • Simulation • Training • Virtual reality • Patient safety Technical skills • Nontechnical skills

---

Key Points
- Traditional models of surgical apprenticeship are no longer fit for purpose.
- Reduced working times are placing surgical trainees under increasing pressure.
- Minimally invasive urological surgery requires high levels of technical and nontechnical skill.

S. Arora, B.Sc.(hons), MBBS, MRCS • S. Undre, MBBS, FRCS, Ph.D. • R. Kneebone, Ph.D., FRCS, FrCGP(✉)
Departments of Surgery and Cancer, Imperial College,
Praed Street, London W2 1NY, UK
e-mail: r.kneebone@imperial.ac.uk

H.R.H. Patel, J.V. Joseph (eds.), *Simulation Training in Laparoscopy and Robotic Surgery*,   31
DOI 10.1007/978-1-4471-2930-1_4, © Springer-Verlag London 2012

- Rapid technological advances require surgeons to gain new skills throughout their careers.
- Recent developments in simulation offer realistic settings for learning and assessment.
- Virtual reality simulators can provide high levels of engagement.
- Technical and nontechnical skills can be measured using validated assessment tools.
- Simulation is used by many high-risk, safety-critical industries for team training.
- Simulation can be used to provide training in technical and nontechnical skills for urologists.
- Simulation training may improve patient safety.

Introduction

The past 10 years have seen profound changes in the delivery of health care and training for urologists. Since the publication of the Institute of Medicine's report, "To err is human," [1] there has been an unprecedented focus upon quality of care [2]. Further studies on both sides of the Atlantic have confirmed that approximately 10% of patients in hospital suffer from an adverse event caused by the care they receive rather than the illness itself [3, 4]. Not surprisingly, the training of clinicians has been called into question. In the United Kingdom, training programs have been dramatically revised under "Modernising Medical Careers" with the emphasis being upon progress based upon demonstrating competency [5]. This has made training of urologists more transparent and accountable but has significantly shortened the time available to train [5]. Training time has been further reduced by the introduction of the European Working Time Directive (EWTD) which states that, as of August 2009, no clinician should work more than 48 h/week. As a result, the opportunities for trainee urologists to learn their skills through experience in the operating room have greatly diminished.

Against this backdrop, technology continues to advance rapidly, bringing major patient benefits. The advent of minimally invasive surgery and robotics has led to reduced postoperative pain, shortened hospital stay, and faster return to normal activity. However, for the operating urologist, the picture is not so simple. These new technologies have brought with them a whole new set of difficulties and challenges [6]. These include the loss of tactile feedback from tissues, the counterintuitive use of instruments due to the fulcrum effect, using a 2D screen to "look at" a 3D field and issues with hand-eye coordination [7]. Significant learning curves to master these techniques reflect the considerable time investment required [8, 9]. Patient safety requirements and ethical considerations in an adversarial medicolegal milieu do not allow for the practice of these skills on real patients. This makes the need for alternative training environments imperative [10]. This chapter explores simulation as an environment for minimally invasive surgery (MIS) training, focusing on its application to urology.

Simulation in Health Care

Simulation offers a promising arena for training complementary to clinical practice [11]. It provides the urologist with the opportunity to learn in a safe, controlled environment—at their own pace and without risk to patients [12]. Evidence suggests that skills acquired in the simulated environment may transfer to the clinical setting [13], making the training potential highly desirable in complex urological procedures. Urology as a speciality lends itself to simulation training as a large number of index procedures are carried out endoscopically. Procedures such as resection of bladder tumors, prostates, and endoscopic stone procedures have been traditionally taught using synthetic models but can now be more realistically taught using high-fidelity virtual reality (VR) simulators.

Incorporation of simulation into educational programs has become increasingly commonplace across a range of domains, both for experiential learning and assessment [14]. Examples include aviation training using flight simulators for pilots [15] and training exercises for the military [16, 17].

Within the health-care domain, although anesthesiologists have paved the way for the integration of simulation into training [18], surgery in general has been slower to adapt. Reasons include high costs and lack of validation of the simulators for teaching the specific task. These issues are slowly beginning to be resolved with further research on validation [19] and the introduction of cheaper, mobile solutions making the benefits of simulation more widely available [20, 21].

However, for simulation to be integrated into any training curriculum, it must be shown that it is effective (i.e., learning objectives are met) and efficient (i.e., minimization of costs and time taken to achieve proficiency) [22]. Strategic planning is thus required to take full advantage of simulation-based learning. Currently, however, there seems to be "little awareness of the substantive and methodological breadth and depth of educational science in this field" [13]. Although simulation does provide trainees with new educational opportunities [23], its potential cannot be fully tapped until the comprehensiveness of its possibilities is appreciated. Simulation can be used to provide training in many of the factors required to produce a competent urologist [24]. Several models of competency have been proposed including those by the ACGME [25], CanMEDS [26], and (within the United Kingdom) by the ISCP [27]. Regardless of which model is utilized, the possibilities of simulation for MIS training for urologists can be broadly categorized into two main domains—technical and nontechnical skills training.

Simulation for Technical Skills Training

Mastering the technical skill of doing a procedure is crucial to any craft specialty, and urology is no exception. Almost half of all adverse events result from the failure of the surgeon's technical skill [4], making this a key determinant of performance and outcome. Within urology, simulation to learn the technical skills for MIS is particularly valuable at the following stages of training:

Basic tasks, where the opportunity to train by experience is decreasing. Traditionally, this individual learning of basic techniques such as cystoscopy has taken place in surgical skills workshops using synthetic and animal-based tissues. More recently, VR simulators are being used to provide training in basic skills (e.g., the Uro Mentor™ Simbionix USA Corp, URO Mentor, Simbionix Ltd., Lod, Israel). Watterson et al. assessed 20 novice trainees for the ability to perform basic uretero-scopic tasks on the Uro Mentor and found that simulator training resulted in quicker training without prior expertise in the procedure [28]. Furthermore, the Uro Mentor has demonstrated excellent construct validity, making it a useful assessment and feedback tool for trainees [29].

High-risk tasks, where the traditional master-apprentice model (MAM) training poses an unacceptable risk to patients. VR simulators in the past 5–10 years are increasingly being used to train surgeons in minimally invasive techniques [30]. Examples include laparoscopic nephrectomy, laparoscopic radical prostatectomy, and more recently robot-assisted procedures including prostatectomies and cystectomies. An example of simulation for complex procedures is provided by Sethi et al., who used a simulator mimicking the da Vinci robot to perform complex oncological procedures such as radical prostatectomy, showing good face and content validity with the Mimic dV-Trainer [31].

Crisis management tasks, where the skills required to deal with a crisis in theater may never be acquired or practiced due to their rare occurrence. Examples include crises such as uncontrolled hemorrhage or cardiac changes leading to a cardiac arrest which would involve not just the surgeons but the entire team. Undre et al. provided a model for such crisis simulation training and assessed the feasibility of using this for training and feedback [32]. Scenarios can be varied, and different surgical simulators or synthetic models can be utilized to simulate uncontrolled bleeding from a transurethral resection of prostate (TURP) or even a TUR syndrome which, although rare events, are potentially catastrophic and require apt crisis management skills. Traditional training provides little opportunity to experience, much less to master these events, and there is considerable variability in individual trainee's skills in dealing with such events.

Simulation can compensate for such heterogeneous experience by ensuring that each trainee attains specified training objectives. This focus on simulation for training in technical skills of MIS has highlighted the science of skills assessment. The use of a global rating scale to assess technical skills (objective structured assessment of technical skills or OSATS) has been applied to urological procedures such as cystoscopy and ureteroscopy [33]. Several assessment methods including the structured observation of skills [34] and motion analysis using tools such as ICSAD (Imperial College Surgical Assessment Device) [35] have been developed. Studies validating urological simulators have also been carried out in an attempt to enhance training [28].

However, although studies have demonstrated the ability of training on a simulated model to improve real performance on patients, there remains a lack of integration of simulation-based training into daily practice [36]. One explanation of this may be that a more realistic type of training focusing upon the wide array of technical and nontechnical skills required of a urologist may be needed to increase face value and therefore uptake of simulation.

Nontechnical Skills Training

Technical skills are undoubtedly important in a practical speciality such as urology, but nontechnical skills are often the root cause of many adverse events in health care and therefore should not be undervalued [3]. Any experienced surgeon realizes that the skills required for effective performance in urology extend beyond individual technical abilities [24]. These "nontechnical skills" refer to a set of behaviors and skills that complement a surgeon's manual dexterity. They can broadly be categorized into two main domains—cognitive and behavioral. Cognitive skills are those that pertain to how and what a surgeon thinks as they perform a procedure. Examples include situation awareness, decision making, and management of stress. Behavioral skills relate to how a surgeon acts or behaves in theater in relation to those around him. This includes the surgeon's communication, teamwork, and leadership skills [37].

An example of nontechnical skills in urology is provided in a study by Clarke et al. [38], who investigated how consultant urologists make treatment decisions about (hypothetical) patients with prostate cancer. They found that even within the consultant grade, there were significant inconsistencies in the treatment recommendations offered.

Effective communication and teamwork are other key nontechnical skills which optimize patient outcomes. In the context of laparoscopic urology, these skills are particularly important for safe surgery. With regard to this, our research group has developed and validated the Observational Teamwork Assessment for Surgery© (OTAS©) tool. This provides a comprehensive assessment and evaluation of teamwork and communication in the OR. It consists of two parts: a teamwork task checklist, filled in by a surgeon, and a set of behavioral ratings, completed by psychologist. Behavior ratings are produced separately for the surgical, anesthetic, and nursing sub-teams that comprise a full OR team. A specific version of this tool has been created and tested within the urology operating theater [39, 40]. In this study, 50 urological procedures were observed using OTAS including both laparoscopic (e.g., cystoscopy, transurethral resection of the prostate) and open (e.g., circumcision and orchidectomy) cases. Anesthetists' and nurses' behavioral ratings were highest for cooperation and lowest on communication; surgeons' ratings had a similar pattern, but their scores were significantly lower in the postoperative phase. Importantly, this study also demonstrated the feasibility and reliability of measuring teamwork in urological surgery.

Nontechnical skills are also particularly required to manage the complex, dynamic, and often stressful environment of the urology operating theater. This is illustrated in another study carried out by our research group, where we measured the distractions and disruptions to the operating urologist in 30 procedures (including laparoscopic) [41, 42]. The study found that the rate of visibly distracting events was 0.45/min—i.e., one distraction every other minute of the procedure. Furthermore, someone walked into or out of the OR every minute of the procedure. Not surprisingly, operative time was found to increase by an average 5.66 min as a result of the disruptions.

Managing an environment such as that described above, while remaining focused to perform the procedure safely, requires high levels of nontechnical skill. So how can these skills be acquired? Unlike other safety-critical industries such as aviation and the military, the importance of teamwork within surgery has often received scant attention in the past. While pilots and army personnel practice with simulation in the form of crew resource training to minimize adverse events [43], nontechnical skills are not addressed within the surgical curricula, leaving most urologists to develop these skills on an ad hoc basis. This is neither safe nor effective.

Using simulation to provide training similar to that used in aviation could help to minimize the potential for error in urological teams [44]. For example, a simulated operating theater could be used to provide an environment in which to practice the response to crisis scenarios without jeopardizing patient safety [45]. This is illustrated in a study by Gettman et al. who used high-fidelity simulation for teaching and assessing teamwork, communication, and laparoscopic skills to urology residents in a simulated operating room. They developed various scenarios related to laparoscopic procedures such as insufflator failure and carbon dioxide embolism leading to eventual patient death [46]. Although such catastrophic events are extremely rare, trainee urologists need to be equipped with the skills to handle them. Simulation provides a powerful opportunity for trainees to learn about these rare but crucial situations in a safe but realistic setting. Although research in this field is still only preliminary, early evidence suggests that such simulation-based programs can help meet the requirements for ACGME core competencies. Standardization of learning experiences and training is another benefit conferred by simulation-based programs. Simulation can thus be used to provide training in basic, high-risk, and crisis management tasks that may improve surgeons' technical and nontechnical performance and ultimately, patient care in urological surgery.

Summary

Urological surgery requires a combination of technical and nontechnical skills. Rapid advances in technology, coupled with radical changes to traditional work patterns, mean that trainees can no longer learn the skills they require through clinical experience alone. Simulation offers an attractive adjunct. Physical and virtual reality simulators can allow surgeons to gain a range of skills and experience while protecting real patients from harm.

References

1. Kohn LT, Corrigan J, Donaldson MS, editors. To err is human: Building a safer health system. Washington, D.C.: National Academy Press; 2000.
2. Department of Health. High quality care for all: NHS Next Stage Review final report 2008.
3. Vincent C, Neale G, Woloshynowych M. Adverse events in British hospitals: preliminary retrospective record review. BMJ. 2001;322(7285):517–9.
4. Gawande AA, Thomas EJ, Zinner MJ, Brennan TA. The incidence and nature of surgical adverse events in Colorado and Utah in 1992. Surgery. 1999;126(1):66–75.
5. Tooke J. Aspiring to excellence: final report of the independent inquiry into modernising medical careers. London: MMC Inquiry; 2008.
6. Belcher E, Arora S, Samancilar O, Goldstraw P. Reducing cardiac injury during minimally invasive repair of pectus excavatum. Eur J Cardiothorac Surg. 2008;33(5):931–3.
7. Aggarwal R, Grantcharov TP, Darzi A. Framework for systematic training and assessment of technical skills. J Am Coll Surg. 2007;204(4):697–705.
8. Aggarwal R, Grantcharov TP, Eriksen JR, et al. An evidence-based virtual reality training program for novice laparoscopic surgeons. Ann Surg. 2006;244(2):310–4.
9. Grantcharov TP, Bardram L, Funch-Jensen P, Rosenberg J. Learning curves and impact of previous operative experience on performance on a virtual reality simulator to test laparoscopic surgical skills. Am J Surg. 2003;185(2):146–9.
10. Arora S, Aggarwal R, Sevdalis N, et al. Development and validation of mental practice as a training strategy for laparoscopic surgery. Surg Endosc. 2010;24(1):179–87.
11. Arora S, Sevdalis N, Nestel D, Tierney T, Woloshynowych M, Kneebone R. Managing intraoperative stress: what do surgeons want from a crisis training program? Am J Surg. 2009;197(4):537–43.
12. Kneebone RL, Nestel D, Vincent C, Darzi A. Complexity, risk and simulation in learning procedural skills. Med Educ. 2007;41(8):808–14.
13. Issenberg SB, McGaghie WC, Petrusa ER, Lee Gordon D, Scalese RJ. Features and uses of high-fidelity medical simulations that lead to effective learning: a BEME systematic review. Med Teach. 2005;27(1):10–28.
14. Kneebone R, Aggarwal R. Surgical training using simulation. BMJ. 2009;338:b1001.
15. Helmreich RL. On error management: lessons from aviation [see comment]. BMJ. 2000;320(7237):781–5.
16. Flin R, O'Connor P, Crichton M. Safety at the sharp end: a guide to non-technical skills. Aldershot: Ashgate; 2008.
17. Arora S, Sevdalis N. HOSPEX and concepts of simulation. J R Army Med Corps. 2008;154(3):202–5.
18. Holzman RS, Cooper JB, Gaba DM, Philip JH, Small SD, Feinstein D. Anesthesia crisis resource management: real-life simulation training in operating room crises. J Clin Anesth. 1995;7(8):675–87.
19. Carter FJ, Schijven MP, Aggarwal R, et al. Consensus guidelines for validation of virtual reality surgical simulators. Simul Healthc. 2006;1(3):171–9.
20. Kneebone R, Arora S, King D, et al. Distributed Simulation – widening access to immersive training for clinical skills. Med Teacher. 2010;32(1):65–70.
21. Paige JT, Kozmenko V, Yang T, et al. High-fidelity, simulation-based, interdisciplinary operating room team training at the point of care. Surgery. 2009;145(2):138–46.

22. Dankelman J, Chmarra MK, Verdaasdonk EG, Stassen LP, Grimbergen CA. Fundamental aspects of learning minimally invasive surgical skills. Minim Invasive Ther Allied Technol. 2005;14(4):247–56.
23. Kneebone R, Kidd J, Nestel D, Asvall S, Paraskeva P, Darzi A. An innovative model for teaching and learning clinical procedures. Med Educ. 2002;36(7):628–34.
24. Arora S, Sevdalis N, Suliman I, Athanasiou T, Kneebone R, Darzi A. What makes a competent surgeon? Experts and trainees perceptions of the role of a surgeon. Am J Surg. 2009;198(5):726–32.
25. Swing SR. Assessing the ACGME general competencies: general considerations and assessment methods. Acad Emerg Med. 2002;9(11):1278–88.
26. Frank JR, Danoff D. The CanMEDS initiative: implementing an outcomes-based framework of physician competencies. Med Teach. 2007;29(7):642–7.
27. ISCP. Intercollegiate Surgical Curriculum Project. Accessed 6 July 2008.
28. Watterson JD, Beiko DT, Kuan JK, Denstedt JD. Randomized prospective blinded study validating acquistion of ureteroscopy skills using computer based virtual reality endourological simulator. J Urol. 2002;168(5):1928–32.
29. Shah J, Darzi A. Surgical skills assessment: an ongoing debate. BJU Int. 2001;88(7):655–60.
30. Aggarwal R, Moorthy K, Darzi A. Laparoscopic skills training and assessment. Br J Surg. 2004;91(12):1549–58.
31. Sethi AS, Peine WJ, Mohammadi Y, Sundaram CP. Validation of a novel virtual reality robotic simulator. J Endourol. 2009;23(3):503–8.
32. Undre S, Koutantji M, Sevdalis N, et al. Multidisciplinary crisis simulations: the way forward for training surgical teams. World J Surg. 2007;31(9):1843–53.
33. Kishore TA, Pedro RN, Monga M, Sweet RM. Assessment of validity of an OSATS for cystoscopic and ureteroscopic cognitive and psychomotor skills. J Endourol. 2008;22(12):2707–11.
34. Martin JA, Regehr G, Reznick R, et al. Objective structured assessment of technical skill (OSATS) for surgical residents. Br J Surg. 1997;84(2):273–8.
35. Datta V, Chang A, Mackay S, Darzi A. The relationship between motion analysis and surgical technical assessments. Am J Surg. 2002;184(1):70–3.
36. Sutherland LM, Middleton PF, Anthony A, et al. Surgical simulation: a systematic review [see comment]. Ann Surg. 2006;243(3):291–300.
37. Yule S, Flin R, Paterson-Brown S, Maran N. Non-technical skills for surgeons in the operating room: a review of the literature. Surgery. 2006;139(2):140–9.
38. Clarke MG, Wilson JR, Kennedy KP, MacDonagh RP. Clinical judgment analysis of the parameters used by consultant urologists in the management of prostate cancer. J Urol. 2007;178(1):98–102.
39. Undre S, Healey AN, Darzi A, Vincent CA. Observational assessment of surgical teamwork: a feasibility study. World J Surg. 2006;30(10):1774–83.
40. Undre S, Sevdalis N, Healey AN, Darzi A, Vincent CA. Observational teamwork assessment for surgery (OTAS): refinement and application in urological surgery. World J Surg. 2007; 31(7):1373–81.
41. Healey AN, Primus CP, Koutantji M. Quantifying distraction and interruption in urological surgery. Qual Saf Health Care. 2007;16(2):135–9.
42. Primus CP, Healey AN, Undre S. Distraction in the urology operating theatre. BJU Int. 2007;99(3):493–4.
43. Helmreich RL, Merritt AC, Wilhelm JA. The evolution of Crew Resource Management training in commercial aviation. Int J Aviat Psychol. 1999;9(1):19–32.
44. Coxon JP, Pattison SH, Parks JW, Stevenson PK, Kirby RS. Reducing human error in urology: lessons from aviation. BJU Int. 2003;91(1):1–3.
45. Moorthy K, Munz Y, Forrest D, et al. Surgical crisis management skills training and assessment: a simulation[corrected]-based approach to enhancing operating room performance. Ann Surg. 2006;244(1):139–47.
46. Gettman MT, Karnes RJ, Arnold JJ, et al. Urology resident training with an unexpected patient death scenario: experiential learning with high fidelity simulation. J Urol. 2008;180(1):283–8.

Chapter 5
Value of Virtual Reality in Medical Education

Amina A. Bouhelal, Hitendra R.H. Patel, and Bijendra Patel

Abstract Surgical training has, for the most part, remained relatively stagnant for a significant length of time. The "see one, do one, teach one" methodology, based within the Halstedian apprentice-type framework, has, until recently, stood the test of time. In this chapter, we discuss the need to enhance the medical education in general and surgical training in particular by embracing simulation. We discuss the necessity for change, and we present the advantages gained by adopting simulation as new novel way to cope with the revolutionized field of surgery in the era of minimally invasive surgery.

Keywords Simulation • Virtual reality • Medical education • Surgical training Minimally invasive surgery

A.A. Bouhelal, MBBS, M.Sc. (✉)
London Surgical Academy, Cancer Institute, Barts
and The London School of Medicine and Dentistry,
Charter House Square, London EC1M 6BQ, UK
e-mail: amina.bouhelal@hotmail.com

H.R.H. Patel MD, PhD
Department of Urology and Endocrine Surgery, University Hospital North Norway,
Breivika, Tromsø N-9038, Norway
e-mail: hrhpatel@hotmail.com

B. Patel, MBBS, MS, FRCS(Ed), FRCS(Gen.Surg)
Department of Upper GI Surgery, Barts Cancer Institute
and Royal London Hospital, Queen Mary University of London,
Charterhouse Square, Barbican, London EC1M 6BQ, UK

H.R.H. Patel, J.V. Joseph (eds.), *Simulation Training in Laparoscopy and Robotic Surgery*,   39
DOI 10.1007/978-1-4471-2930-1_5, © Springer-Verlag London 2012

Key Points

Simulation

- Overcoming the human factor and ensuring excellence of care and patient safety
- Standardized, safe training environment
- Equalized training opportunities and exposure among trainees
- Objective evaluation and focused individualized assessment
- Repletion toward proficiency and permission to fail
- Critical thinking, decision making, and self-reflection
- Enhancing learning curves and evidence-based developed training schemes
- Filling the gap between the theoretical knowledge and practical experience
- Instrument development and testing and research
- Medical care cost control by minimizing complication

Tell me and I will forget; show me and I may remember; involve me and I will understand.
Confucius, 450 BC

Introduction

Surgery was not always the prestigious specialty with the mystique around it that is today. When the British surgeons attempted to separate surgery from the barbers' practice by requesting the establishment of the Royal College of Surgeons in 1797, Lord Thurlow, the Lord Chancellor of England at the time, spoke his or her famous words: "there is no more science in surgery than in butchery" [1, 2].

Surgical training has been long dependent on apprenticeship. Where surgeons were to be trained on actual patients in the operating theaters, learning in the job was the only way to learn. Apprenticeship largely relies on unpredictable clinical nature of case load, the experience of the instructor, his or her interest, and subjectivity. The prolonged operating time and alarming complication rates were not the only impediments. The exposure varies greatly among different trainees, and standardization remains simply not possible. Despite the crucial long-played role of surgical apprenticeship, it is being increasingly subjected to inadequacy and progressively failing in meeting the new field demands.

The apprenticeship is largely subjective, time-consuming, and cost-ineffective.

Guaranteed equal exposure among trainees is not feasible, and achieving the balance between mentoring and patient care in an increasingly busy schedule can be overwhelming for the mentors, with one responsibility fulfilled at the expense of the other, especially with the decreased number of faculty pursuing academic careers and many of them leaving for private practice.

Aspiring for better health care compels the medical society in general and the surgical society in particular to pursue novel alternatives to ensure the continuity of training quality, equality, and excellence of patient care.

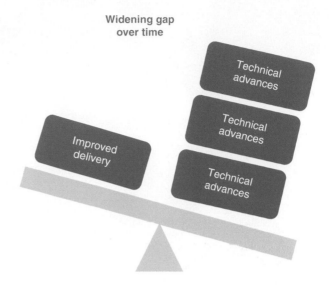

Fig. 5.1 The current mismatch between the technical advances and the delivery of care

Many great innovations were introduced to the surgical field in the last century. Minimally invasive surgery, for example, is no longer a luxury; it has become rather the present era and pressing reality of surgery, imposing the challenge of formulating and exploring novel approaches to enhance the surgical education.

Developing effective alternatives in order to supplement the trainees with the fundamentals of the practice is the current quest of the surgical society, especially when surgeons are required to learn more and perform further in shorter period of time. Beside sound knowledge, superior reasoning, efficient decisiveness, and effective communication along with skills competency, a wide variety of whole new expertise has become indispensable with the shift to minimally invasive surgery.

Dimensional awareness, eye-hand coordination, and depth perception, among many other skills, are utterly necessary.

A skillfully performed operation is 75% decision making and 25% dexterity [3]. In minimally invasive surgery, one can hypothesize that dexterity plays an even more crucial role. The global technological development necessitates the need to enhance delivery and therefore training methods, and since our decisiveness is greatly dependent on our acquired knowledge, previous exposure, and experience, practice indeed makes perfect. And what can be of superior value in our learning journey than our own mistakes? (Fig. 5.1)

The capability to readily imitate and reproduce clinical scenario, with sufficient sensitivity to differentiate subject skills, estimate competency, and utilize quantitative metrics, when possible, to evaluate performance, is what medical education needs, and that is exactly where simulation presents itself as the desperately needed alternative with undeniable impact and indisputable advantages.

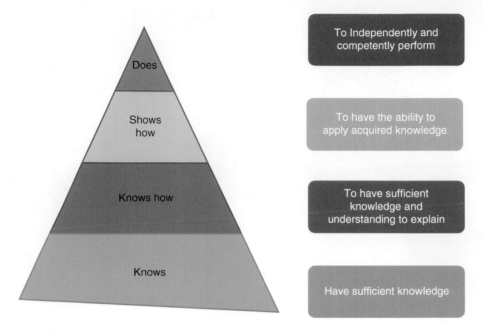

Fig. 5.2 The effectiveness of simulation in comparison to other teaching methods

Simulation in Medical Education

Simulation in the medical education is revolutionizing the practice, with many centers and professionals adapting and adopting simulation in all its various forms. Simulation can be considered the answer to minimally invasive surgery training. Most of the commercially available simulators provide the reliability of testing, and offer a much-needed property, by introducing objectivity to long subjectivity-dependent field (Fig. 5.2).

The advantages of simulation extend beyond empowering the training schemes with safe environment for skill acquisition; it incorporates the effectiveness of communication skills teaching, interpersonal relation development, and teamwork exercise coaching. How can we justify the rather dramatic shift in the medical education, explain the need to change, and justify the expenses? Why simulation?

Value of Simulation

Patient Care and Safety

"Do no harm" the patient care and safety are the center of attention. However, in the United States, 99,180 actual deaths and $8.9 billion represent the possibly avoidable deaths and associated costs [4], not to mention the disabilities and loss of function and work hours. The impact on the economy is massive.

Although many factors are implicated in such high life loss figures, the failure to perform at high competency level due to undertraining and lack of exposure can be held liable for the unnecessary and largely avoidable complications.

Simulation has proved to be a viable option; practicing on patients presents an increasingly growing ethical, moral, and medicolegal responsibility, jeopardizing not only patient care and safety but the quality of teaching and training. The availability of the simulation makes the learning and the practicing of the generic procedures, and skills required to an indentified proficiency level possible. After which the trainee can safely proceed to perform in real-life scenarios.

The Transformation of the Educational Experience

Ericsson and Reznick accentuate that exposure and repetition rather than innate ability is what determines the skill acquisition and efficiency of training [5].

Simulation provides a secure, safe, and standardized educational environment in which trainees are offered equal opportunities and variable clinical scenarios; the training does not need to depend on how and when the cases present themselves, and the training is not restricted by the meticulous amalgamation of the instructor schedule, patient willingness, and availability or the rarity of the cases. Training time can be allocated and protected to secure the educational experience, resulting in a more productive training generated by eliminating external factors and keeping interference to minimum.

How can simulation be more efficient than traditional methods?

- Overcoming the human factor
- The opportunity to apply knowledge
- Skills acquisition and repetition toward proficiency, with the ability to alter and adjust the difficulty level
- The ability to set learning objectives and training schedule
- Independency of the training from cases' availability or concerns over patient safety
- Devotion of training irrespective to the work service and mentor schedule
- The luxury of repetition and permission to fail
- Possibility of critical thinking, decision making, and self-reflection
- Lavishness of focused learning at the individual's own pace and learning needs with best usage of exposure hours
- Objective assessment of performance and building of confidence
- Immediate feedback and possibility of tackling the weaknesses and augmenting the strength points
- Gaining clinical experience and learning by exposure, self-reflecting and personal intuition development, and the exchange of knowledge with colleagues
- Developing the ability of teamwork playing and effective management and leadership
- New equipment testing
- Development and research

With effective exposure and focused personalized training, the ability of the trainees and their competency can be drastically enhanced. The trainee can be prepared to deal with what he or she has yet to encounter [3, 6, 7].

Cost-Effectiveness

The cost of medical errors the United States economy endured in 2008 was $17.5 billion [8].

Convincing the medical education society with the educational value and cost-effectiveness of simulators is one of the main obstacles standing in the way of integrating simulation into the medical training. The evidence needs to be compelling in order to advocate the expenses. We should consider and compare the simulator cost as an initial investment to the value that will be gained. When dealing with potentially life-threatening situations, the cost of simulator training is well worth the investment.

Most of the commercially available simulators in their various types and categories are designed to withstand the extensive handling and use; they are easy to operate and survive the repetitive utilization, which in turn minimizes the expenses. Although the economical status can and usually interferes with any progress, one should not forget that unlike many other fields in which we can bear and support the cuts and delay the changes, the medical field is not one of these fields; we simply cannot afford the cost of lost lives.

Many clinicians still assume that the expenditure of simulation is unjustifiable. However, studies showed that the overall cost is in fact decreased due to reduced training hours, instructor time, and complication cost which result from insufficient training and premature patient practice [8–10].

Laparoscopic Cholecystectomy Skills Acquisition and Procedural Proficiency in Novices Using Virtual Reality

In our study researching procedural proficiency and skill acquisition in novices using virtual reality, the initial data collected demonstrated significant improvement, especially in total time and path length.

Abstract

Aim

Our study objectives are to investigate the time and attempts needed by novices to reach proficiency in laparoscopic cholecystectomy using virtual reality and to help add to the literature toward establishing an evidence-based training curriculum.

Methods

Following open advertising, 30 novices were recruited to participate in our study. The novices were trained on nine basic tasks, four procedural tasks, and full laparoscopic cholecystectomy on a high-fidelity, commercially available Simbionix Lap Mentor VR simulator. An adapted and adopted training curriculum was used. The performance of experienced laparoscopic surgeons was taken as a benchmark for proficiency level, and learning curve analysis was done [11].

Results

A total of 30 novices successfully completed the training curriculum, and their performance was analyzed. The basic tasks 5 and 6 and procedural tasks 3 and 4 were included in the curriculum, as well as full laparoscopic cholecystectomy procedure.

All participants reached proficiency level, however, at different paces. In basic task 5, the average time taken to finish the task decreased from 2:35 min to 1:35 min in mean total simulator time of 12:49 min with average number of trials of 7.3.

In basic task 6, participant's performance illustrated a speedy progress with average time taken to finish the task decreasing from 2:19 to 1:17 min in mean total simulator time of 12:33 min with average number of trials of 7.2.

In procedural task 3, participant's average time taken to finish the task decreased from 7:48 to 4:00 min in mean total simulator time of 26:42 min with average number of trials of 5.33.

In procedural task 4, participant's average time taken to finish the task decreased from 6:44 to 4:00 min in mean total simulator time of 27:40 min with average number of trials of 5.2.

In the Full Procedural LC, participant's average time taken to finish the task decreased from 6:44 to 4:00 min in mean total simulator time of 27:40 min with average number of trials of 5.2. With number of trials required to achieve proficiency ranging between 3 and 21, establishing the fact that certain individuals require longer time and number of repetitions, which is firmly reflective to reality where trainee learning scales differ greatly (Fig. 5.3).

Conclusion

All our study participants reached proficiency level, however, with a range of time, number of movements, and total path length, which is very reflective to reality. It is our hope to help establish time and number of attempt for novices in training to achieve laparoscopic cholecystectomy curriculum proficiency in virtual reality–based training.

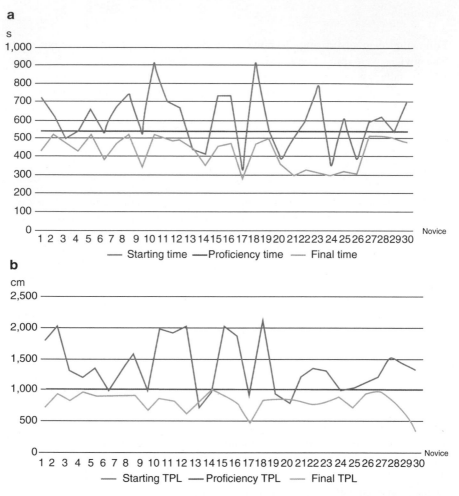

a

s

b

cm

Fig. 5.3 (**a**) Time: Novices' first and final attempts vs. proficiency. An illustrated comparison between the initial and final performance time of the novices to the proficiency level. (**b**) Total path length: Novices' first and final attempts vs. proficiency. An illustrated comparison between the initial and final total path length of the novices to the proficiency level. (**c**) Number of movements: Novices' first and final attempts vs. proficiency. An illustrated comparison between the initial and final number of movements of the novices to the proficiency level

c

Movement

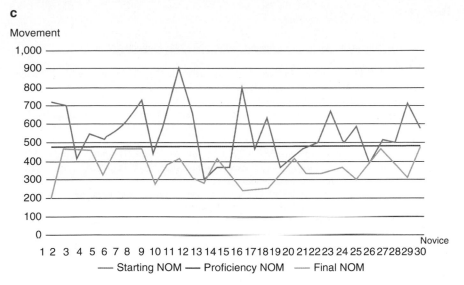

— Starting NOM — Proficiency NOM   — Final NOM

Fig. 5.3 (continued)

Summary

"Simulation is an educational technique that allows interactive and at times immersive activity by recreating all or part of a clinical experience without exposing patients to the associated risks" [7].

Simulation is offering the medical education with long-needed solutions to ensure and secure the quality of teaching and patient care and safety. It is not whether simulation is effective or not, its effectiveness is well established, and the evidence is irrefutable. It is whether we are ready to embrace and use the technology or not.

> *The reasonable man adapts himself to the world; the unreasonable one persists in trying to adapt the world to himself. Therefore, all progress depends on the unreasonable man.*
> *George Bernard Shaw*

References

1. Shaw AB. Benjamin Gooch, Eighteen-Century Norfolk Surgeon. Med Hist. 1972;16(1): 40–50.
2. Moynihan BT. The Approach to Surgery Delivered at the Opening of the Session at King's College Hospital Medical School. Br Med J. 1951;2(4735):848.
3. Müller-Tomfelde C. Interaction sound feedback in a haptic virtual environment to improve motor skill acquisition. In: Barrass S, Vickers P, eds. *10th Meeting of the International Conference on Auditory Display* (ICAD 2004); Sydney, NSW. ICAD; 2004. CD ROM. ISBN: 1741080487 (CD), 1741080622 (Web).
4. HealthGrades Seventh Annual Patient Safety in American Hospitals Study, March 2010. Available at: http://www.healthgrades.com/media/DMS/pdf/PatientSafetyInAmerican-HospitalsStudy2010.pdf. Accessed 24 Oct 2011.
5. Resnick L, Hall MW. Principles of Learning for Effort-based Education. In: Principles of Learning: Study Tools for Educators (CD-ROM), Version 3.0. University of Pittsburgh; 2003.
6. Murray C, Grant MJ, Howarth ML, Leigh J. The use of simulation as a teaching and learning approach to support practice. Nurse Educ Pract. 2008;8(1):5–8.
7. Maran NJ, Glavin RJ. Low- to high-fidelity simulation – a continuum of medical education? Med Educ. 2003;37 Suppl 1:22–8.
8. Van den Bos J, Rustagi K, Gray T, Halford M, Ziemkiewicz E, Shreve J. The $1.71 billion problem: the annual cost of measurable medical errors. Health Aff (Millwood). 2011;30(4): 596–603.
9. Okuda Y, Bryson EO, DeMaria Jr S, Jacobson L, Quinones J, Shen B, Levine AI. The utility of simulation in medical education: what is the evidence? Mt Sinai J Med. 2009; 76(4):330–43.
10. Aucar JA, Groch NR, Troxel SA, Eubanks SW. A review of surgical simulation with attention to validation methodology. Surg Laparosc Endosc Percutan Tech. 2005;15(2):82–9.
11. Aggarwal R, Crochet P, Dias A, Misra A, Ziprin P, Darzi A. Development of a virtual reality training curriculum for laparoscopic cholecystectomy. Br J Surg. 2009;96(9):1086–93.

Chapter 6
The MIMIC Virtual Reality Trainer: Stepping into Three-Dimensional, Binocular, Robotic Simulation

Steven M. Lucas and Chandru P. Sundaram

Abstract The dramatic increase in the number of robotic surgeries performed has prompted a need for more rigorous robotics training during or after residency, yet training in robotic surgery requires the instructing surgeon to partially relinquish control of the procedure, which makes this training difficult. The MIMIC® virtual reality trainer, MdVT (Mimic Technologies Inc., Seattle, WA), provides a means for trainees to acquire skills prior to entering the operating room. In this chapter, the features of the MdVT as well as the available training exercises are reviewed. Preliminary face, content, and construct validity of the trainer has been established using basic exercises and will be discussed. Finally, the future development of this robotic trainer in terms of further establishing validity and creating new training exercises will be summarized.

Keywords Robotic surgery • Virtual reality simulation • Three-dimensional simulation • Performance scoring • Validation

> **Key Points**
> * MdVT has binocular vision and a three-dimensional virtual reality surgical field.
> * The two haptic endowrists track grip closure and rotational and translational movement in all three axes.
> * The parts of the virtual console reflect those of the dVSS.

S.M. Lucas, M.D. • C.P. Sundaram, M.D. (✉)
Department of Urology, Indiana University,
535 N. Barnhill Dr., Suite 420, Indianapolis, IN 46202-5289, USA
e-mail: sundaram@iupui.edu

H.R.H. Patel, J.V. Joseph (eds.), *Simulation Training in Laparoscopy and Robotic Surgery*, 49
DOI 10.1007/978-1-4471-2930-1_6, © Springer-Verlag London 2012

- Training exercises available fall into three categories: (1) targeting, (2) object manipulation, and (3) suturing.
- Metric scoring provides immediate feedback and includes time, economy of motion, accuracy, and force as main types of information.
- Three recent studies have demonstrated face, content, and construct validity for the MdVT.
- One recent study demonstrates criterion validity.
- Suturing on the MdVT is difficult and is a target for improvement.
- Future research will focus on the criterion validity of the MdVT.
- Future developments include addressing surgical "bottlenecks" and simulating actual surgical scenarios.

Introduction

Following the first robotic prostatectomy performed in 2000 [1, 2], the use of robotics has rapidly grown, with two hospitals per week purchasing a surgical robot by 2006 [3]. With the increased use of this minimally invasive technique, the procedures performed have also become more complex. This has necessitated the development of a structured robotic curriculum, including skills training and simulation. Conventional operating room instruction for minimally invasive surgery is difficult, as the technique implies there is minimum access to the surgical field. This requires the instructing physician to relinquish control of the operative field to the trainee. The beginner, as per the theory of motor learning purported by Fitts and Posner, is often in the cognitive phase of learning, where movements are erratic, broken into distinct steps, and inefficient, which often leads to the conclusion of the operating room lesson [4].

To make learning more efficient, simulators have been added to many surgical curricula, including both inanimate (bench) simulators and virtual reality simulators. Inanimate simulators are less expensive and can help develop basic tasks from camera movement to suturing, which can translate to improved performance in live surgical scenarios. However, they require time to evaluate progress and are limited in their ability to create realistic surgical scenarios. This may lead to a decreased usefulness as the trainee progresses. Virtual reality simulators can be very expensive, up to $300,000 for the more complex machines [5, 6]. However, they offer a means of accurately assessing performance with little effort by the instructor or trainee [7]. Construct validity has been reported in several different laparoscopic virtual reality simulators [5, 8, 9]. Haptic feedback, which may allow trainees more rapid acquisition of laparoscopic skills, is diminished, but even newer trainers have attempted to recreate this [10]. Virtual reality simulators also have the potential to reflect more realistic surgical scenarios. Training on these simulators has been shown to improve performance in live surgical scenarios [11, 12]. Though current literature cannot validate superiority of either inanimate or virtual reality simulators, improvement in virtual reality simulators may eventually allow trainees to perform several virtual cases prior to performing a live laparoscopic case in the operating room.

Although there are currently several virtual reality simulators for laparoscopy, developing virtual reality simulators for robotic surgery has proven to be more difficult. The simulation of three-dimensional, binocular vision and the increased degrees of freedom have been the main obstacles to overcome. Thus, many institutions employ "dry" lab training sessions in which trainees may perform tasks on inanimate models, using the robot at times when it is not being used for surgery or a robot specifically for training, both of which can have substantial costs. Recently, a three-dimensional virtual reality simulator named MIMIC dV-Trainer (MdVT, Mimic Technologies Inc., Seattle, Washington) has been developed. In the following chapter, we review the different parts, training exercises, literature assessing validity, and future developments of the MdVT.

The MIMIC Simulator: The Parts

The MIMIC mantis consists of one haptic interface, developed in 2004, and the Mantis Duo has two haptic interfaces, developed in 2006. The Mimic Mantis Duo (Fig. 6.1) haptic interfaces have master grips consisting of the two straps and a closeable grasper that simulate the grips found on the surgeon console of the da Vinci Surgical System® (dVSS, Intuitive Surgical, Sunnyvale, CA). The master grips are connected to a gimbal endowrist which allows for rotational freedom of motion as well as bending similar to that found on the wrist of the dVSS instruments. The two gimbals are attached to the platform of the simulator via a total of eight tension cables. Through the cables, data is sent to an onboard 520 mHz

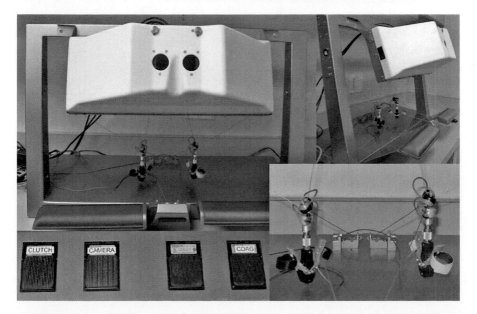

Fig. 6.1 Photograph of the MdVT shows the binocular eye piece, workspace range in the front and side views. The master grips with endowrist gimbals and the clutching and cautery pedals are highlighted

processor and translated into the simulated environment via the host computer. The cables provide 7 degrees of tracking, including grip closure, and translation and rotation about the x, y, and z axes. In addition, the interface provides force feedback in these three axes. The workspace is 79 cm in width, 52.2 cm in height, and 39.4 cm in depth. The cables allow for a maximum force of 15.2 N and a continuous force of 3.3 N at the center of the workspace [13].

Two docking platforms, which are used for calibration of the gimbals, are located within the workspace. An armrest, similar to that found on the dVSS console, is also provided. The stereoscope provides binocular vision of a virtual three-dimensional environment. It is connected to the host computer via a 100 Mbit Ethernet interface and allows for haptic updates at a rate of 1,000 Hz, with an accuracy of 0.3 degrees and 0.016 mm. Also connected to the interface is a pedal platform consisting of four pedals including the camera clutch, instrument clutch, and two coagulation pedals [13].

Training Exercises

The MdVT offers training tasks that range in difficulty, including camera movement and object targeting, object manipulation and cautery, and suturing (Fig. 6.2). Many of these training exercises are adaptations of standardized training exercises first developed from inanimate models [6]. These exercises are arranged into beginner,

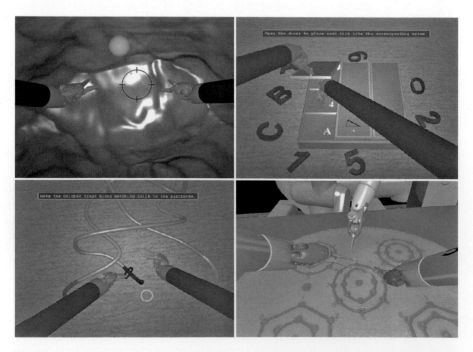

Fig. 6.2 Example exercises available for the Mimic trainer: Object Targeting, Advanced Letter Board, Ring Pass, and Dots and Numbers (Courtesy MIMIC Technologies, Inc., used with permission)

intermediate, and advanced curricula. Newer interfaces allow one to customize the curricula to include the exercises of his/her own choosing. The simplest example of a targeting exercise is camera targeting of an object, which requires the trainee to locate objects placed in various locations outside of the view of the simulator, by clutching the camera and the instruments. Tasks of object manipulation can include transferring pegs to a board, placing letters on a board, running a ring along a tube, or cutting. Suturing exercises include tasks such as suturing sponges or patterns that reflect live surgical scenarios.

The exercise tasks are evaluated with the metrics provided by the MdVT program. Immediate metric feedback on errors and overall performance may enhance the acquisition of skills [7]. The automated MdVT metrics score trainees in three different aspects, which are modified to have relevance to each task. The first of these, targeting, scores whether a desired object or view is touched, passed, or centered. The second, efficiency, includes task time, economy of motion, instrument collisions, time spent outside of view, dropped objects, and master workspace range. Master workspace range evaluates a trainee in the ability to use the clutch, thereby keeping the instrument controls in the center of the console. Finally, force can also be evaluated with respect to force applied onto the instrument and strain placed on the tissue.

Validation

In order for a simulator to be effective as a training tool, it must be demonstrated to be representative of what it is simulating (content validity), realistic and easy to use (face validity), and distinguish different levels of surgical experience (construct validity), and it must be shown to have criterion validity [14]. Criterion validity includes both the demonstration that the training performance of the simulator is better than the current standard (concurrent validity) and the ability to predict future performance (predictive validity). While recent research has demonstrated the face, content, and construct validity, further research on criterion validity is needed.

Initial evaluation of the MdVT was performed at the AUA in 2007. Lendvay et al. demonstrated construct validity among 4 experts and 11 novices. In this study, the subjects removed, transferred, and replaced rings on cones. The same exercise was performed on the dVSS and the MdVT. Relative to the novices, the experts performed better in terms of time, economy of motion, and time instruments spent out of the center. The subjects, when surveyed, rated both the dVSS and the MdVT as acceptable means of training [15].

Further validation by Sethi et al. compared the performance of 5 experts and 15 novices on the MdVT. Construct validity was assessed using three different exercises: Ring and Cone, String Walk, and Letter Board. Although the experts performed all tasks faster and more efficiently, statistically significant improvements in time to completion and time instruments spent out of view were seen only in the Letter Board. Statistical differences may have been muted as the tasks performed on the MdVT were developed to imitate the tasks performed already in a dry lab curriculum by the novices. The experts generally approved of the practice format, relevance, and

Table 6.1 Summary of validation studies for the Mimic trainer

Series	Number of subjects	Type of validation	Exercises studied	Significant metrics
Lendvay et al. [15]	4 experts 11 novices	Construct, face, content	Peg Transfer	Time, economy of motion, time out of center
Sethi et al. [16]	5 experts 15 novices	Construct, face, content, task load	Ring and Cone, Ring Walk, Letter Board	Time, time out of center
Kenney et al. [17]	7 experts 19 novices	Construct, face, content	Dots and Numbers suturing, Suture Sponge, Peg Board, Pick and Place	Time, total motion, time out of center, number successful, missed, unattempted targets
Lerner et al. [18]	12 MdVT trainees 11 dVSS trainees	Predictive, concurrent	Targeting, Ring Walk, Pick and Place, Letter Board	Time and accuracy comparison on dVSS

usefulness of the MdVT as a training tool (giving scores 4–5 out of 5 on the Likert scale). Face validity was assessed by both the novices and the experts. Ease of use and realism of the MdVT in terms of its visual and hardware aspects averaged 4 of 5 on the Leikert scale (5 being "very easy/real"). The precision of movement, however, had less approval, with a mean score of "average ease of use/realism" (3 of 5). The experts demonstrated a lower task load than the novices in all dimensions, but this was statistically significant only for mental demand and effort to complete the task [16].

A final study of the content, face, and construct validity compared 19 novices and 7 experts. The suturing aspect of the MdVT was assessed. The experts performed better in the metrics of total instrument motion, task time, time spent out of the center of the workspace, and number of successful, missed, and unattempted targets, in the Dots and Numbers (a circle with suture targets inside and outside the circle), Suture Sponge, Peg Board, and Pick and Place. Although the study confirmed that most users of the MdVT find it realistic and useful, the suturing aspect received a mean "slightly unacceptable" score (3 out of 6 on a Leikert scale) [17].

The consistency of results of the three studies demonstrates that the MdVT has reasonable construct validity and is perceived to be realistic to most users. However, suturing is one area that requires improvement.

While the construct validity has been demonstrated, less research is available on the criterion validity. Lerner et al. have recently compared the performance of participants training on the MdVT (12) with those training on the dVSS (11). In this study, both groups performed baseline tests on the dVSS, including object manipulation exercises, pattern cutting, and a suture with knot-tying exercise. The MdVT group then trained on the MdVT, while the dVSS group trained on the dVSS. A final session on the dVSS was scored for all subjects. Relative to the dVSS group, the MdVT group demonstrated greater improvement on the pattern cutting and peg placement exercises. While the dVSS group showed significant improvement in the knot-tying exercise, the MdVT group demonstrated improvement that was not statistically significant for this exercise [18]. Table 6.1 summarizes validation studies for the MdVT. Further research should include corroboration of the findings by Lerner et al. and assessment of how training on the MdVT will impact performance on live surgical procedures. Similar research conducted for standard laparoscopic virtual reality simulators demonstrates improved performance in real surgical scenarios following training on different virtual reality trainers [11, 12, 19–21].

Future Direction

Although the MdVT trainer provides a unique simulation of three-dimensional robotic surgery, it does have limitations, which require improvement. Suturing and tying is one such limitation, as Keeney et al. demonstrated that content validity for this aspect is rated as "slightly unacceptable" by expert surgeons [17]. The needle, suture, and response of tissue to manipulation were deemed to not be realistic. This has already been improved upon in the laparoscopic virtual reality simulators [20, 22].

Another area in which improvement is sought is in the force aspect of the trainer. The tissue response to manipulation by the operator "strain" and the force applied to the instrument by the operator and the environment are haptic limitations shared by many virtual reality simulators. The MdVT does have some haptic feedback with translational and rotational movement. It has been shown that the addition of haptic feedback onto a laparoscopic virtual reality simulator enhanced the acquisition of laparoscopic skills in novices [10].

Collaboration between MIMIC and Intuitive Surgical could result in simulation software being used by the surgeon on the da Vinci Surgical System's console but without the patient side cart and the robotic arms. This would eliminate all the hardware drawbacks associated with the simulator without the need to use the patient side cart and the instruments. Further software development will allow the complete realization of the potential of robotic surgical simulation.

Other developments are being made in making the exercises more procedure based. This will initially focus on the challenging or "bottleneck" portions of the procedure (i.e., urethrovesical anastomosis, nerve-sparing, or pyeloplasty anastomosis; Fig. 6.3).

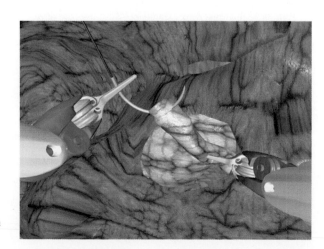

Fig. 6.3 Future direction: addressing surgical "bottlenecks." A pyeloplasty anastomosis is shown (Courtesy MIMIC Technologies, Inc., used with permission)

These can then be developed into entire procedures, with conditions that could change in accordance with the progression of the surgery. Finally, mapping actual patient data into a simulated program would allow practice of a certain aspect of the procedure prior to completing it in a patient.

Summary

The MdVT provides a platform for virtual reality robotic training in a three-dimensional format. It currently offers training through a series of tasks, which can be evaluated by metric analysis to discriminate the expert from the novice. While training on the virtual reality trainer improves performance of tasks on the trainer, demonstrating improved performance on the dVSS or in live surgical scenarios is not yet complete. Future developments of this simulator will include improved simulation of suturing and procedure-based exercises.

References

1. Binder J, Kramer W. Robotically-assisted laparoscopic radical prostatectomy. BJU Int. 2001;87:408–10.
2. Pasticier G, Rietbergen JB, Guillonneau B, et al. Robotically assisted laparoscopic radical prostatectomy: feasibility study in men. Eur Urol. 2001;40:70–4.
3. Steinberg PL, Merguerian PA, Bihrle 3rd W, et al. A da Vinci robot system can make sense for a mature laparoscopic prostatectomy program. JSLS. 2008;12:9–12.
4. Reznick RK, MacRae H. eaching surgical skills—changes in the wind. N Engl J Med. 2006;355:2664–9.
5. Maithel S, Sierra R, Korndorffer J, et al. Construct and face validity of MIST-VR, Endotower, and CELTS: are we ready for skills assessment using simulators? Surg Endosc. 2006;20: 104–12.
6. Scott DJ, Bergen PC, Rege RV, et al. Laparoscopic training on bench models: better and more cost effective than operating room experience? J Am Coll Surg. 2000;191:272–83.
7. Snyder CW, Vandromme MJ, Tyra SL, et al. Proficiency-based laparoscopic and endoscopic training with virtual reality simulators: a comparison of proctored and independent approaches. J Surg Educ. 2009;66:201–7.
8. McDougall EM, Corica FA, Boker JR, et al. Construct validity testing of a laparoscopic surgical simulator. J Am Coll Surg. 2006;202:779–87.
9. Woodrum DT, Andreatta PB, Yellamanchilli RK, et al. Construct validity of the LapSim laparoscopic surgical simulator. Am J Surg. 2006;191:28–32.
10. Panait L, Akkary E, Bell RL, et al. The role of haptic feedback in laparoscopic simulation training. J Surg Res. 2009;156:312–6.
11. Andreatta PB, Woodrum DT, Birkmeyer JD, et al. Laparoscopic skills are improved with LapMentor training: results of a randomized, double-blinded study. Ann Surg. 2006;243:854–60.
12. Lucas SM, Zeltser IS, Bensalah K, et al. Training on a virtual reality laparoscopic simulator improves performance of an unfamiliar live laparoscopic procedure. J Urol. 2008;180: 2588–91.
13. Mimic Technologies, Inc. http://www.mimc.ws. Accessed 5 October 2009.

14. McDougall EM. Validation of surgical simulators. J Endourol. 2007;21:244–7.
15. Lendvay TS, Casale P, Sweet R, et al. VR robotic surgery: randomized blinded study of the dV-Trainer robotic simulator. Stud Health Technol Inform. 2008;132:242–4.
16. Sethi AS, Peine WJ, Mohammadi Y, et al. Validation of a novel virtual reality robotic simulator. J Endourol. 2009;23:503–8.
17. Kenney PA, Wszolek MF, Gould JJ, et al. Face, content, and construct validity of dV-trainer, a novel virtual reality simulator for robotic surgery. Urology. 2009;73:1288–92.
18. Lerner MA, Ayalew M, Peine WJ, Sundaram CP; Does Training on a Virtual Reality Robotic Simulator Improve Performance on the *daVinci*® Surgical System? J Urol. 2010, in press.
19. Cosman PH, Hugh TJ, Shearer CJ, et al. Skills acquired on virtual reality laparoscopic simulators transfer into the operating room in a blinded, randomised, controlled trial. Stud Health Technol Inform. 2007;125:76–81.
20. Halvorsen FH, Elle OJ, Dalinin VV, et al. Virtual reality simulator training equals mechanical robotic training in improving robot-assisted basic suturing skills. Surg Endosc. 2006;20:1565–9.
21. Seymour NE, Gallagher AG, Roman SA, et al. Virtual reality training improves operating room performance: results of a randomized, double-blinded study. Ann Surg. 2002;236.458–63.
22. McDougall EM, Kolla SB, Santos RT, et al. Preliminary study of virtual reality and model simulation for learning laparoscopic suturing skills. J Urol. 2009;182:1018–25.

Chapter 7
Laparoscopic Cholecystectomy Skills Acquisition and Procedural Proficiency in Novices Using Virtual Reality

Amina A. Bouhelal, Hitendra R.H. Patel, and Bijendra Patel

Abstract *Background*: Training within a proficiency-based virtual reality curriculum has been proven to be an effective enhancement to supplement the conventional surgical training schemes that have been stagnant for a significant period of time. In our study, we investigated the time and attempts needed by novices to reach proficiency in laparoscopic cholecystectomy using virtual reality to help add to the literature toward establishing a training curriculum.

Methods: Thirty-two novices were prospectively and randomly recruited to participate in our study. Novices were trained on 9 basic tasks, 4 procedural tasks, and full laparoscopic cholecystectomy on a high-fidelity, commercially available virtual reality simulator, Lap Mentor, Simbionix. A validated training curriculum was used where the performance of experienced laparoscopic surgeons was used as a benchmark for proficiency level.

Results: A total of 30 novices successfully completed the training curriculum and reach proficiency level, expectedly at different paces, which is very reflective of reality.

Conclusion: It is feasible to methodically design VR-based training curriculums and scientifically introduce VR to training schemes, providing a safe environment for training novices toward attaining procedural proficiency and assuring an objective assessment and quality of aptitude using expert performance as a benchmark.

A.A. Bouhelal, MBBS, M.Sc.(✉)
London Surgical Academy, Cancer Institute, Barts and The London School of Medicine and Dentistry, Charter House Square, London EC1M 6BQ, UK
e-mail: amina.bouhelal@hotmail.com

H.R.H. Patel MD, PhD
Department of Urology and Endocrine Surgery, University Hospital North Norway, Breivika, Tromsø N-9038, Norway
e-mail: hrhpatel@hotmail.com

B. Patel, MBBS, MS, FRCS(Ed), FRCS(Gen.Surg)
Department of Upper GI Surgery, Barts Cancer Institute
and Royal London Hospital, Queen Mary University of London,
Charterhouse Square, Barbican, London EC1M 6BQ, UK

Keywords Virtual reality • Simulation • Training • Proficiency • Novices

Key Points
- Virtual reality is a feasible and important enhancement to surgical education.
- Validated curriculums with proficiency criteria are essential for surgical training.
- Virtual reality training and the simulator metric assessment will introduce the field long missing objective evaluation.
- It is viable to construct and scientifically allocate protected training time for surgical trainees and create a more constructive training.
- The value of virtual reality can extend to incorporate in-practice surgeons for performance evaluation, periodic assessments, and revalidation.

Introduction

Surgical training has long relied on the Halstedian apprentice-type framework. As the case load increases and the working hours decreased, along with the ever-escalating operation complexity, apprenticeship is no longer a valid choice to guarantee the supply of qualified safe surgeons the specialty needs.

Simulation in its various forms has long played a very essential role in filling the gap between the theoretical knowledge and operation room experience, and virtual reality (VR) is no exception. The emerging evidence supporting VR as an effective novel method in medical education is irrefutable.

About 10–15% of the adult Western population has gallstones. Between 1% and 4% become symptomatic each year. In the United Kingdom, 50,000 cholecystectomies are performed annually of which 70–90% are carried out laparoscopically [1].

Before VR can be fully integrated into the training schemes, validated curriculums need to be produced along with clear idea about the number of attempts and simulator time needed.

Our study using a validated published procedural specific, laparoscopic cholecystectomy curriculum [2], investigated the attempts and time needed by a novice to reach proficiency.

Recruitment and Methodology

A novice surgeon in our study was defined as a medical student, with no previous exposure to laparoscopy, or experience in simulation. Thirty-two students were randomly recruited; 30 finished the study curriculum.

Inclusion Criteria

- Candidate interested and keen to commit.
- Medical background.
- Basic knowledge of relevant hepatobiliary anatomy; however, detailed unified explanation was provided to all participants to eliminate any potential bias.
- No previous exposure to laparoscopy, contact limited to observing.
- No previous exposure to Lap Mentor™ simulator or any form of surgical simulation VR or otherwise.

Exclusion Criteria

- Laparoscopic exposure beyond observation.
- Any form of laparoscopic training, VR or otherwise, e.g., box trainer.
- Failure to finish the study curriculum.

Lap Mentor™ Platform

The LAP Mentor simulator is one of the best commercially available simulators in the market, and among the highly effective platforms accessible, with its advanced design that is both sophisticated and user-friendly.

In addition, the haptic interface on the LAP Mentor offers enhanced tactile feedback, performance, and reliability.

The realistic visualization of the human anatomy created by the Lap Mentor is exceptional and gives a very representative recreation of the intra-abdominal cavity and organs.

Methods of Training

Training started by an induction session in which all trainees were provided with one-to-one explanation of the study and explanatory demonstration of the simulator and the tasks by same instructor to eliminate any potential bias.

A standardized comprehensive explanation was given using unified visual aids and covered the following:

- General explanation about the study and what is expected from the novices; however, all trainees were kept blind to the proficiency criteria.
- Overview about the simulator, Lap Mentor™.
- Demonstration on how to utilize the simulator and how to handle and change instruments.

- Anatomical knowledge required for laparoscopic cholecystectomy including and not limited to the anatomy of hepatobiliary system and the organs visualized.
- General possible problem and troubleshooting.

A validated training curriculum from Aggarwal et al. [2] was used for training. Explanation and demonstration was carried out by single specific instructor, who was available at all time with the participants. All participants were kept blind to the proficiency criteria and the required aptitude level.

The simulator used in the study is the same used in the validated curriculum.

All participants received induction sessions for all 9 basic tasks and 4 procedural tasks, and the full laparoscopic cholecystectomy; however, for training sessions and assessment against proficiency, only basic tasks 5 and 6 and procedural tasks 3 and 4 along with standard anatomy full laparoscopic cholecystectomy were used.

For the full laparoscopic cholecystectomy procedure, in addition to the objectivity of assessment provided by the metric feedback of the simulator and validated proficiency level provided by the validated used curriculum, a modified version of the General Surgical Skills Global Rating and Operation Specific Surgical Skills Global Rating were used to assess proficiency.

Data Collection

The Lap Mentor™ simulator automatically provides a metric feedback after each task; the data were gathered and analyzed. The General Surgical Skills Global Rating and Operation Specific Surgical Skills Global Rating was completed by the observing instructor for the full laparoscopic cholecystectomy and used for evaluation toward proficiency.

Participants Demographics

A total of 32 students were recruited, 30 successfully finished the study curriculum, and their performance data was included.

Results

A total of 30 novices successfully completed the training curriculum. Expectedly at different paces, this is very reflective of reality.

In basic task 5, the average time taken to finish the task after training was 1:21 min in mean total simulator time of 12:49 min in 7.3 attempts.

In basic task 6, the average time taken to finish the task after training was 1:16 min in mean total simulator time of 12:19 min in 7.2 attempts.

In the procedural task 3, the average time taken to finish the task after training was 3:43 min in mean total simulator of 26:42 min in 5.33 attempts.

In the procedural task 4, the average time taken to finish the task after training was 3:45 min in mean total simulator of 27:40 min in 5.2 attempts.

In the full procedural laparoscopic cholecystectomy, the average time taken to finish the task after training was 7:10 min in mean total simulator time of 30:03 min in 3.4 attempts (Fig. 7.1).

The total simulator time and the range of number of trials needed by participants to reach proficiency level varied from one participant to another; again, this stresses the utility of the standardized and individualized training VR-based teaching provides.

The time measured and analyzed in our study refers to the period of time participant spent working on the simulator, from the start of the task to its end, and it does not include the break times or the time to organize, load, and prepare the tasks.

Discussion

Using a validated curriculum with proficiency criteria is of great value toward a safe and structured training that assures the efficacy and quality of training, along with the immense magnitude of objective assessment.

All our participants demonstrated remarkable improvements throughout the steps of the study curriculum, while all 30 of them reached proficiency in all curriculum steps, by examining both the performance of the participants in the basic procedural tasks, and the full procedure and analyzing their performance, we put emphasis on the importance on using proficiency criteria, not due to the great value of maintaining the objectivity of the training only, but also the importance of training toward a target, being one of the most vital factors.

It is essential, however, to allow time to plateau phase in future VR-based training studies which in turn mean longer training time and more simulator time.

Although this time may not be considered a reflective value in reality, it can, however, give an idea about the probable needed time.

Conclusion

All novices reached proficiency level and completed the study curriculum, despite the variation in all metrics among the participants, making the possibility of an established procedural training curriculum possible.

With predetermined proficiency criteria, novices are trained and assessed objectively toward competency, at their own pace.

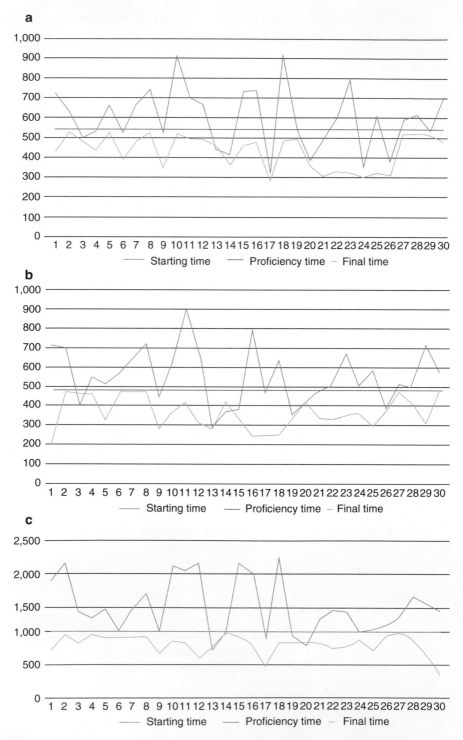

Fig. 7.1 Graphic representations of the novices' initial and final attempts to complete a full laparoscopic cholecystectomy compared against the expert performance. (**a**) Time, (**b**) number of movements (NOM), (**c**) total path length (TPL) (in cm)

VR-based training is of great implications and can certainly add to the surgical training in its current form if implemented correctly. VR is the pillar of many other industries and has been repeatedly proven useful; perhaps surgical education can benefit from VR to broaden the horizons of not only patient care and excellency of education but for revalidation of in-practice surgeons and as a tool for surgical trainees selection process in an increasingly competitive field that continues to put great emphasis on the theoretical knowledge while neglecting the innate surgical talent, simply because the surgical society lacks the tools to objectively assess it.

Although the change may not be immediate, it will certainly be indispensable in the near future.

References

1. Gurusamy K, Samraj K, Gluud C, Wilson E, Davidson BR. Meta-analysis of randomized controlled trials on the safety and effectiveness of early versus delayed laparoscopic cholecystectomy for acute cholecystitis. Br J Surg. 2010;97(2):141–50.
2. Aggarwal R, Crochet P, Dias A, Misra A, Ziprin P, Darzi A. Development of a virtual reality training curriculum for laparoscopic cholecystectomy. Br J Surg. 2009;96(9):1086–93.

Chapter 8
Lesson Learnt from the Military Surgeons Using Simulation in Trauma Surgery

Simon S. Fleming and John-Joe Reilly

Abstract The low exposure of many trauma team members to severe trauma under-lines the need for alternatives to "learning by doing" when the "doing," in the early stages, involves a trauma patient. This is unacceptable with today's patient safety requirements and often unobtainable with modern surgical training. Equally in the dynamic, high-pressured environment of managing trauma patients, the risk of errors occurring and miscommunications is rife. Management of a trauma patient, whether in the emergency department, operating theater, or intensive care unit, relies on the performance of the team as a whole and as such will only work with both effective technical skills but also nontechnical skills such as communication or delegation.

The evidence shows that when a trauma team is trained using simulation, there are significant improvements in the quality of teamwork and a reduction in clinical errors in the trained groups.

Keywords Trauma • Simulation • Military • Surgery • War

S.S. Fleming, MBBS(Lond), MRCS(Eng), M.Sc.(Surg)(✉)
Queen Mary University of London,
Old Anatomy Building Charterhouse Square,
London, Great Britain EC1M 6BQ, UK and

London Surgical Academy, Cancer Institute, Barts & The London Medical School
and NHS Trust, London, UK
e-mail: simonsfleming@doctors.org.uk

J.-J. Reilly, B.Sc.(Hons), GiBiol, Ph.D., DIC, BMedSci(Hons), BM, BS
Academic Department of Military Surgery and Trauma,
Royal Centre for Defense Medicine, University Hospital Birmingham,
Birmingham B152TH, UK

H.R.H. Patel, J.V. Joseph (eds.), *Simulation Training in Laparoscopy and Robotic Surgery*, 67
DOI 10.1007/978-1-4471-2930-1_8, © Springer-Verlag London 2012

Key Points
- Trauma is not something in which one can guarantee real-life experience.
- There is no risk to patients as errors can occur safely.
- Management of routine events and procedures can be practiced and improved.
- Realistic setting is provided.
- Scenarios can be created to provide (time) flexible and specific learning opportunities.
- Training is easily reproducible.
- Learning is experiential, participatory, and enjoyable.
- Immediate feedback is possible.
- There is a risk that the technology overshadows educational principles.
- Training builds on both technical and nontechnical skills such as team working and communication.

Introduction

Simulation is, in itself, nothing new. From the first moment when the doctors and surgeons of days gone by practiced on animals and cadavers before being allowed to practice their art, simulation was playing a role in preparing us for what is to come. However, trauma, and simulating trauma, brings its own unique set of challenges and motivations. There are limited opportunities for clinicians to gain the necessary experience needed to effectively manage trauma unless working in a busy trauma environment and not all of us can be so "lucky." Trauma is, by its very nature, an unexpected event. A trainee may work an entire rotation and never deal with a major trauma patient, with all of the technical and nontechnical skills (such as communication, dynamic decision making, situational awareness, and teamwork) that a situation such as that requires. True, there are numerous trauma courses available, such as the Acute Trauma Life Support Course (ATLS), Specialty Skills in Emergency Surgery and Trauma (SSEST), and Definitive Surgical Trauma Care (DSTC/DSTS), but even they rely on simulation, moulage, and human patient simulators (HPS) for their teaching and assessments. When it comes to dealing with trauma, simulation is often the best way to prepare oneself for the real thing [1].

Surgeons must be very careful
When they take the knife!
Underneath their fine incisions
Stirs the Culprit—Life!
Emily Dickinson

Surgical training has, up until rather recently, remained relatively stagnant for a significant length of time. The "See One, Do One, Teach One" methodology, based

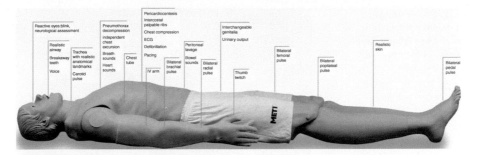

Fig. 8.1 CAE Healthcare METI human patient simulator (Courtesy CAE Healthcare; used with permission)

within the Halstedian apprentice-type framework, has stood the test of time. But with the need to train surgeons while still keeping patient safety at the forefront, things had to change [2]—but how? Is it still appropriate for the first experience a surgeon has of being involved in the care of a trauma casualty to be their first trauma patient? It was only through looking toward other professional areas such as airline pilots or even piano players that it was discovered that to become what the lay person might consider an "expert" required 10,000 h or 10 years of practice [3], and that to maintain this level of skill required one not to simply be "in the job" but in fact a new concept in surgical training—to take part in deliberate practice [4–6], which is extremely difficult in the trauma setting where unlike many other clinical settings, one cannot be guaranteed exposure to it on a regular basis. Thus, the trainee must be motivated, recognizing that their patient exposure and time in theaters will be far less with today's training frameworks and demands for a "senior lead" service, and that their chances to just "get on with it" as of old are no more [7]. Yet, even with motivation, one can never simply hang around a resuscitation bay, waiting for that perfect polytrauma to rill through the doors; service provision and real life get in the way.

The answer seems to be simulation training, and the acceptance of simulation training by all facets of the medical community is on the rise [8]. This is because managing a trauma patient, whether in the emergency department or the operating theater, is not simply a one-man show. It is a team effort, with numerous people playing numerous roles, all while using different equipment—in theory, a recipe for chaos. Miscommunication has been widely cited as contributing to things gone awry, often during the times when it is most vital that things run smoothly [9, 10]. Simulation has been shown to be a way around this; since time immemorial, military forces have used drill and exercises to prepare both individual soldiers and units for war [11], and this is no different to what we might consider "simulation training."

Whether using full patient; high-fidelity simulators, which can go into shock and exsanguinate at the push of a button (Fig. 8.1), actors covered in makeup and special effects (Fig. 8.2) (there are numerous companies that not only supply actors for moulage and simulation, but these can include amputees so that no imagination is

Fig. 8.2 A simulated
traumatic amputation
(Courtesy Action Amps
(ACS) Ltd.; used with
permission)

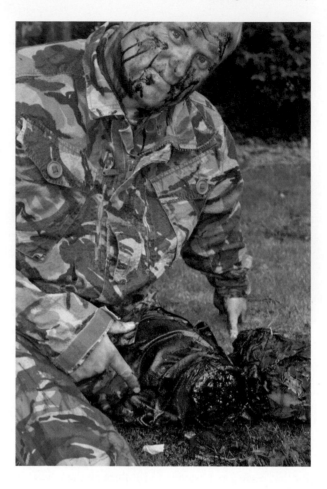

required! [12]), box trainers, virtual reality trainers, or animal/cadaveric material, there are numerous methods by which one can prepare for the management of a trauma patient without laying hands on an actually critically unwell person. It is true though that the whole experience has an air of the theatrical about it and a degree of "suspended disbelief" is required to maximally utilize simulation though most manage easily.

With all this in mind, it is clear that there is a role for simulation within trauma training—allowing for safer, less judgmental, more time efficient, training. Numerous studies [13] have been performed across the numerous facets of medicine where simulation training is used and have shown, time and again, assuming the simulation training is used appropriately (Table 8.1), then both the cognitive and affective (e.g., leadership/teamworking skills or perhaps even the appreciation of other's anxiety in a stressful situation) skills of the trainee will be improved [14, 15]. So, the advantages are clear—safer for the patient, allowing surgical trainers to reduce the likelihood of error and improve clinical outcome as well as giving the

Table 8.1 Appropriate simulation criteria

Constructive feedback given
The opportunity to deliberately practice
Valid training scenarios
Integrated within a curriculum
Clear learning outcomes defined
A variety of conditions and situations possible
A range of difficulty
Controlled setting

trainee an opportunity to train free of inherent ethical issues found in "practicing on patients" and the time constraints faced by all surgeons nowadays. Yet, as with all things, there are drawbacks to training by surgical simulator. Surgical training must include appropriate grounding in theory and in technical skills. There is no use learning how to "ace the simulator," like a child with a computer game they play all the time, rather than with an understanding of the anatomy and pathophysiology relevant to that particular case! The other significant pitfall is the reliance on simulation as the be all and end all of training. More and more in the literature, studies are showing that to effectively train a surgeon, one must move aware from a reliance on technology and see it as a tool within the wider scope of surgical education that surgical training is not simply training an automaton to perform a technical task with the minimum number of errors but instead to educate holistically through a partnership with education and clinical practice [16, 17]. A leading exponent of simulation training has himself noted this issue and said "simulators are only of value within the context of a total educational curriculum, and the technology must support the training goals" [18]. It is vital that the technology becoming available improves the quality of education, rather than simply giving students access to a newer, "shinier" mode of accessing it!

Yet, we must always be mindful, and as Kneebone states [19], "above all, simulation must take its place as one component of a larger picture, supporting and supported by research, technology, clinical practice, professionalism and education."

Military Trauma Training

The defining feature of military trauma simulation training is that it is designed to emulate realistically as possible situations that medical personnel and soldiers will experience while deployed in theaters of operations. The rationale being that the closer the training is to reality, the easier it will be to successfully implement, when faced with real-life casualties. Simulation training takes place at many different levels:

Macrolevel—A field hospital deploying into a theater of operations will first have to undertake a HOSPEX (hospital exercise). A replica of the field hospital is built, and the staff will undergo a rigorous training program and final exercise to ensure that the staffs are fully prepared for their role. This exercise involves all elements of the hospital including Medical Emergency Response Teams (MERT) and Close Support Medical Group, along with senior military commanders. The HOSPEX is designed to train people for anything they may have to deal with in their theater of operations, including mass casualty incidents.

Microlevel—Individuals are trained to varying degrees depending on their defined role. Every British soldier is taught basic first aid as part of their infantry training; however, at section and company level, there are specifically trained medics with more advanced skills. The current gold standard of simulated military trauma training at the moment is the Battlefield Advanced Life Support Course (BATLS) [20]. The BATLS course is an evolving concept based on operational experience and the best available evidence. It uses experienced instructors along with highly realistic simulated casualties to train medics, doctors, and other medical staff in how to deal with trauma injuries that are sustained on the battlefield.

Summary

Work across the spectrum of medical fields has confirmed that the making of errors is a universal phenomenon. It has also shown that this is found at all levels of training but that crucially experience helps to prevent, reduce, and rectify them—and trauma is no different [21, 22].

In a situation such as the traumatically injured patient, where it is recognized that trainees *must* learn but that patient safety demands an already experienced team to manage the patient, simulation training helps facilitate that learning process, while not affecting patient safety. It enhances the acquisition of knowledge and both technical and nontechnical skills, and by providing a realistic environment for training, it facilitates learning by setting it in a relevant clinical context (experiential learning) [23].

It allows all members of the trauma team to experiment with "cause-and-effect" relationships observing realistic responses to treatments given or interventions performed, again, something that is unrealistic in terms of the old "learning on patients" style of training.

As the twenty-first century progresses and patient safety and efficiency become ever more prevalent in our thoughts, more and more, we are going to be taking after the airlines and training in a trauma curriculum incorporating simulation, which is essential if we want to be able to take care of our patients to the best of our ability and in their best interests [24].

References

1. Morey JC, Simon R, Jay GD, et al. Error reduction and performance improvement in the emergency department through formal teamwork training: evaluation results of the MedTeams project. Health Serv Res. 2002;37:1553–81.
2. Smith R. All changed, changed utterly. British medicine will be transformed by the Bristol case. BMJ. 1998;316:1917–8.

3. Small S. Thoughts on patient safety education and the role of simulation. Virtual Mentor. 2004;6:3.
4. Gaba D. Anaesthesiology as a model for patient safety in health care. BMJ. 2000;320:785–8.
5. Ericsson KA. The acquisition of expert performance: an introduction to some of the issues. In: Ericsson KA, editor. The road to excellence: the acquisition of expert performance in the arts and sciences, sports and games. Mahwah: Lawrence Erlbaum Associates; 1996. p. 1–50.
6. Ericsson KA, Krampe RT, Tesch-Romer C. The role of deliberate practice in the acquisition of expert performance. Psychol Rev. 1993;100:363–406.
7. Guest CB, Regehr G, Tiberius RG. The lifelong challenge of expertise. Med Educ. 2001;35: 78–81.
8. Roberts KE, Bell RL, Duffy AJ. Evolution of surgical skills training. World J Gastroenterol. 2006;12:3219–24.
9. Zinn C. 14,000 preventable deaths in Australian hospitals. Br Med J. 1995;310:1487.
10. Schaefer HG, Helmreich RL. The importance of human factors in the operating room. Anesthesiology. 1994;80(2):479.
11. Good ML, Gravenstein JS. Anaesthesia simulators and training devices. Int Anesthesiol Clin. 1989;27:161–8.
12. http://www.actionamps.com/
13. Fletcher G, Flin R, McGeorge P, Glavin R, Maran N, Patey R. Rating non-technical skills: developing a behavioural marker system for use in anaesthesia. Cogn Technol Work. 2004;6: 165–71.
14. Peters JH, Fried GM, Swanstrom LL, Soper NJ, Sillin LF, Schirmer B, Hoffman K. Development and validation of a comprehensive program of education and assessment of the basic fundamentals of laparoscopic surgery. Surgery. 2004;135(1):21–7.
15. Powers KA, Rehrig ST, Irias N, Albano HA, Malinow A, Jones SB, Moorman DW, Pawlowski JB, Jones DB. Simulated laparoscopic operating room crisis: an approach to enhance the surgical team performance. Surg Endosc. 2008;22:885–900.
16. Hoffman HM. Teaching and learning with virtual reality. Stud Health Technol Inform. 2000;79:285–91.
17. Torkington J, Smith SG, Rees BI, Darzi A. The role of simulation in surgical training. Ann R Coll Surg Engl. 2000;82:88–94.
18. Satava RM. Surgical education and surgical simulation. World J Surg. 2001;25:1484–9.
19. Kneebone J. Simulation in surgical training: educational issues and practical implications. Blackwell Med Educ. 2003;37:267–77.
20. Joint Services Publication 570: Battlefield Advanced Trauma Life Support. 4th ed. 2008.
21. DeAnda A, Gaba DM. Role of experience in the response to simulated critical incidents. Anesth Analg. 1991;72:308 15.
22. Byrne AJ, Jones JG. Inaccurate reporting of simulated critical anaesthetic incidents. Br J Anaesth. 1997;78:637–41.
23. Bradley P, Bligh J. One year's experience with a clinical skills resource centre. Med Educ. 1999;33:114–20.
24. Knudson MM, Khaw L, Bullard MK, Dicker R, Cohen MJ, Staudenmayer K, Sadjadi J, Howard S, Gaba D, Krummel T. Trauma training in simulation: translating skills from SIM time to real time. J Trauma. 2008;64(2):255–63; discussion 263–4.

Chapter 9
Clinical and Educational Benefits of Surgical Telementoring

Knut Mague Augestad, Taridzo Chomutare, Johan G. Bellika,
Andrius Budrionis, Rolv-Ole Lindsetmo, Conor P. Delaney and
Mobile Medical Mentor (M3) Project Group[*]

Abstract *Background*: Videoconference technology has substantially improved
making surgical telementoring more feasible. However, evidence of potential
benefits is missing.

[*]Knut Magne Augestad, M.D. (Norwegian Center for Telemedicine and Integrated Care, University
Hospital North Norway, Tromsø, Norway), Taridzo Chomutare, M.Sc. (Norwegian Center for
Telemedicine and Integrated Care and Tromsø Telemedicine Labaratory, University Hospital North
Norway, Tromsø, Norway), Johan Gustav Bellika M.Sc., Ph.D. (Medical Informatics and
Telemedicine Group, Department of Computer Science, University of Tromsø, Tromsø, Norway),
Rolf Ole Lindsetmo M.D., MPH, Ph.D. (Professor and Chief, Department of Gastrointestinal
Surgery, University Hospital North Norway, Tromsø, Norway), Gunnar Hartvigsen Ph.D. (Professor,
Department of Computer Science, Faculty of Science, University of Tromsø, Norway), Per Hasvold
M.Sc. (Research Fellow, Norwegian Centre for Telemedicine and Integrated Care, Tromsø,
Norway), Richard Wootton D.Sc., Ph.D. (Editor in Chief Journal of Telemedicine and Telecare and
Head of Research Norwegian Centre for Telemedicine and Integrated Care, Tromsø, Norway), Stig
Muller M.D., Ph.D. (Consultant, Department of Surgery, University Hospital North Norway,
Tromsø; Norway), Hiten Patel BMSc.Hons, BM, BCh, MRCS, PhD, FRCS (Urol), FRCS (Eng).
(Professor of Surgery & Urology, University of North Norway, Tromsø, Norway), Conor Delaney
M.D., Ph.D. (Professor of Surgical Education and Chief Division of Colorectal Surgery, University
Hospitals Case Medical Center, Cleveland, OH, USA), Alexander Horsch Ph.D. (Professor Institute
for Medical Statistics and Epidemiology, University of Technology, Munich, Germany), Ole Edvard
Gabrielsen M.D. (Consultant, Department of Surgery, Narvik Local Hospital, University Hospital
North Norway), Kim Mortensen M.D., Ph.D. (Consultant, Department of Surgery, University
Hospital North Norway, Tromsø Norway), Sture Pettersen M.Sc. (Head Tromsø Telemedicine
Laboratory, Norwegian Centre for Telemedicine and Integrated Care, Tromsø, Norway)

H.R.H. Patel, J.V. Joseph (eds.), *Simulation Training in Laparoscopy and Robotic Surgery*,   75
DOI 10.1007/978-1-4471-2930-1_9, © Springer-Verlag London 2012

K.M. Augestad, M.D. (✉)
Norwegian Center for Telemedicine and Integrated Care,
University Hospital North Norway, Tromsø, Norway
e-mail: knut.magne.augestad@telemed.no

T. Chomutare, M.Sc.
Norwegian Center for Telemedicine and Integrated Care and Tromsø Telemedicine Labaratory,
University Hospital of North Norway, Tromsø, Norway

J.G. Bellika, Ph.D.
Medical Informatics and Telemedicine Group,
Department of Computer Science, University of Tromsø,
Tromsø, Norway

A. Budrionis, M.Sc.
Norwegian Centre for Integrated Care and Telemedicine, Tromsø, Norway

Department of Computer Science, Carolina State University, USA

R.-O. Lindsetmo, M.D., Ph.D., MPH
Department of Gastrointestinal Surgery, University Hospital North Norway,
Tromsø N-9036, Norway

C.P. Delaney, MB, MCh, Ph.D., FRCSI, FACS, FASCRS
Division of Colorectal Surgery, Department of Surgery,
University Hospitals Case Medical Center, Case Western Reserve University,
11100 Euclid Ave., 44106-5047 Cleveland, OH, USA

Objective: To present evidence of benefits and highlight major barriers, as well as reporting own experience.

Methods: A systematic review was performed; studies were classified as technology-driven, clinical, or educational.

Results: Three hundred and ninety-two surgical procedures were performed by 179 surgeons in 11 surgical specialties. The most common telementored procedure was laparoscopic cholecystectomy (56 cases, 14%), endovascular treatment of aortic aneurysm (48 cases, 12%), and laparoscopic colectomy (24 cases, 6%). One hundred and eleven (27%) cases had a laparoscopic approach; 6 cases (5%) were converted to open surgery. Ten complications (2%) were reported (liver bleeding, trocar port bleeding, bile collection, postoperative ileus, wound infection, serosal tears, iliac artery rupture). Seven surveys (27%) focus on education of surgeons; all these report improved surgical performance. Sixty-three medical students, 48 general surgeons, and 24 surgical residents participated. Telementoring was combined with simulator training in two cases and robotics in three cases. Thirteen surveys (50%) were cross institutional and 7 surveys (27%) were intercountry or intercontinental. Perceived usefulness of surgical telementoring was high among 83% of surgeons; however, only 5 (19%) surveys had a systematic evaluation of surgeon's technology satisfaction.

Conclusion: There is an acceptable rate of conversion and complications. Surgical telementoring is commonly used for education of surgeons and has huge potential to offer patients the best expertise despite long distances.

Keywords Surgical telementoring • Laparoscopy • Telemedicine • Surgical education • Information and computing technology

Introduction

In 1962, Dr. Michael Ellis DeBakey pioneered the field of telemedicine with the first videoconferencing (VC) demonstration of open-heart surgery to be transmitted overseas by satellite [1–3]. Since the 1960s, there has been substantial development in the uses of VC among surgeons [4], including surgical telementoring. Surgical specialists are usually sparsely geographically distributed, and with the predicted shortage of medical professionals, videoconference systems that enable guidance to remote novice surgeons will become increasingly important. The expected result of proper on-site mentoring is improved surgical practice, education, treatment, and postoperative care [5, 6]. Surgical telementoring has been described as a natural fit in surgery [7]; solutions have been demonstrated for laparoscopic surgery [8–10] and in combination with robotic surgery [11–13]. Furthermore, VC has gained increasing popularity in all fields of medicine, especially in education and outpatient treatment of patients [14–17]. Recent developments in information and computing technology (ICT) have led to a renewed interest in the potential of telemedicine to provide new collaborative solutions for surgeons, and recently, a national US research initiative was launched [18]. Little attention has been paid to the clinical benefits of the telemedicine solutions. One criticism found in much of the literature on surgical telementoring is that studies to date have tended to focus on the first level in Friedman's Tower of Achievements [19] (pilot), effectively disregarding the last level (study of effects) where the effect on clinical processes and outcomes are evaluated. Several studies have attempted to provide evidence for cost-effectiveness [20 22] and safety [23–25] of telementoring systems, but there is insufficient data for making claims about clinical and educational outcomes. Previously, we have reported on potential benefits of VC [14] as well as performed comprehensive review on surgical telementoring [26]. The objective of this chapter is to summarize our previous experiences and review [26], characterize successful implementations, and infer future direction of surgical telementoring.

Methods

Details of search methods are presented elsewhere [26]. Main sources were PubMed, Association of Computing Machinery, and Institute of Electrical and Electronics Engineers. After discussion among coauthors, the following combination of search terms was applied: *surgical, telementoring, telesurgical, teleconsultation, laparoscopic,* and *videoconference.*

We included all surveys published from 2000 to 2010. We identified three main categories in the selected surveys:

Clinical aspects refer to whether the paper had a clinical outcome: morbidity, mortality, conversion rate, operation time, length of stay, and surgery on human subjects.

Educational aspects were defined as telementoring with purpose to educate surgeons with focus on the learning curve, trainee satisfaction, and skills assessment.

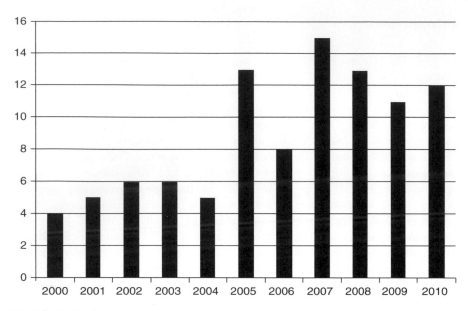

Fig. 9.1 Publication of surgical telementor studies by year. Based on eligible studies assessed for inclusion and exclusion criteria

Technical aspects were defined as papers focusing the technical challenges of telementoring, like bandwidth, video encoding, resolution, delay of voice, and picture.

Results

Twenty-seven papers were included in the final review [11, 27–52]. There was an increasing trend in the number of surveys assessing surgical telementoring (Fig. 9.1). Forty-four percent (12) of studies were located in the United States, followed by Canada with 19% (5), the United Kingdom (3), Italy, Austria, Brazil, Germany, France, and Switzerland (1). According to primary outcome, surveys were classified as clinical (12), technical (15), or educational (7); 7 trials had combination of categories. Three studies had a randomized design [35, 38, 48], and the remaining studies had a prospective or case-case control design. Most studies were classified as Friedman's phase III (80% system installation).

Clinical Aspects

Twenty-three papers reported on clinical outcomes [8, 11, 27–37, 39, 41–45, 49–52]. No clinical outcomes were identified in three papers assessing telementoring via robotics and simulators [38, 47, 48]. There were performed 392 surgical procedures by 179 surgeons. The surveys covered all surgical fields, digestive surgery being the most common specialty (124 cases, 31%). The most common surgical procedure was laparoscopic cholecystectomy (56 cases, 14%), endovascular treatment of aortic aneurysm (48 cases, 12%), and laparoscopic colectomy (24 cases, 6%). One hundred and eleven (27%) cases had a laparoscopic approach, and 6 cases (5%) were converted to open surgery. Ten major complications were reported including liver bleeding, port-site bleeding, bile collection, postoperative ileus, wound infection, serosal tears, and iliac artery rupture (Table 9.1).

Educational Aspects

Seven surveys (27%) reported an educational aspect of their outcome [30, 32, 35, 38, 39, 47, 48]. Two studies involved medical students (63), two surveyed general surgeons (48), and three surveyed surgical residents (24). In all surveys, one mentor was involved. Two surveys combined telementoring with use of surgical simulators. The impact of telementoring on surgical achievement was evaluated by several methods: recognition of anatomical landmarks, "Global Operative Assessment of Laparoscopic Skills," and measurement of task performance (grasping, cutting, clip applying, suturing, economy of movement). All surveys report an expert-novice mentor situation. Three surveys reported mentoring across organizational borders (university hospital, local hospital), and two surveys were intercontinental. Two surveys included use of simulators, and three surveys used robotics (remote camera control or grasper). All surveys report a positive effect of telementoring on surgical achievement (Table 9.2).

Technical Aspects

Nineteen percent (5) of the studies used mobile platforms such as cell phones or personal digital assistants (PDA). None of these were done in a clinical setting, most studies prior to 2006 having only ISDN lines (bandwidth of 512 kbps or less). The popular solution in such circumstances was 4 ISDN lines of 128 kbps each for dual communication lines. After 2006, wireless local area networks (WLAN) show increased popularity as a communication platform. Six studies (23%) specify the video encoding method, and 7 studies (26%) specify video resolution. Eight studies (29%) report specific measurements of video transmission delay, only two solutions to provide a delay within an acceptable range (one-way 250 ms; two-ways: 500 ms). Thirteen studies use telestration, and one study uses mouse pointer. Most studies (73%) use commercial solutions, but in-house developed ($n=5$) and freeware solutions ($n=2$) have also been used (Table 9.3).

Table 9.1 Clinical features of surgical telementoring

Surgical specialty	Procedure	Mentored cases (n=392)	Operative time (min) Mentored	Operative time (min) Not mentored	Complications conversions	Mentor affiliation or location	Number of mentors	Author
Urology	Lap nephrectomy Endoscopic urology	5	NA	NA	None	Expert-resident	NA	Argawal [11]
	Nephrectomy Pelvic node dissection Renal biopsy	14	NA	NA	None	NA	NA	Bauer [28]
	Lap nephrectomy	4	240	225	None	Expert-resident	1	Challacombe [31]
	Lap varicocelectomy Percutaneous nephrolithotomy	2	25	NA	None	Expert-expert	1	Rodrigues Netto [37]
Endocrine	Adrenalectomy	8	NA	NA	Liver bleeding Trochar port bleeding	Expert lap-expert open	1	Bruschi [29]
	Thyroidectomy	25	NA	NA	None	UH-residents	1	Rafiq [39]
	Thyroidectomy	15	NA	NA	None	Expert-expert	NA	Tamariz [49]
Digestive surgery	Lap cholecystectomy	34	NA	NA	Bile leak 1 Conversion	Expert-resident	NA	Byrne [30]
		12	92	94	None	Expert-resident	NA	Sawyer [41]
		10	NA	NA	None	Expert-resident	NA	Parker [51]
	Endoscopic procedures	23	NA	NA	None	NA	NA	Gandsas [35]
	Lap colectomies	4	150	108	Postoperative ileus Wound infection	UH-local	1	Schlachta [42]
		2	150	124	Wound infection Bleeding	UH-local	1	Schlachta [43]
		18	NA	NA	Serosal tears 2 Conversions	UH-local	NA	Sebajang [44]
	Bilateral inguinal hernia	2	105	NA	None	UH-local	1	Rodas [27]
	Lap fundoplication, ventral hernia	19	NA	NA	Hemoperitoneum 2 Conversions	UH-local	NA	Sebajang [45]

Specialty	Procedure				Complications	Relationship		Reference
Emergency medicine	Bovine surgery, heart, lower extremities, head	48		56% improvement speed of completion mentored group	None		NA	Ereso [32]
Neurosurgery	Craniomaxillofacial	50	NA	NA	None	UH-local	NA	Ewers [33]
		6	NA	NA	None	UH-local	NA	Mendez [36]
Gynecology	Lap hysterectomy, explorative lap procedures	20	NA	NA	None	Consultant-resident	NA	Gambadeuro [34]
Pediatric surgery	Lap jejunal polyp Diaphragma hernia Atresia	3	90 30 90	NA	None	Experienced-less experienced	NA	Rothenberg [8]
Vascular surgery	Endovascular treatment aortic aneurysm	48	127	120	Iliac artery rupture 1 Conversion	UH-local	NA	Di Valentino [50]
Orthopedic	Arthroscopic	20	NA	NA	None	Expert-expert	NA	Seemann [52]

There were performed 392 surgical procedures by 180 surgeons. Eleven surgical specialties were represented. The most common surgical procedures were laparoscopic cholecystectomy (56 cases, 14%), endovascular treatment of aortic aneurysm (48 cases, 12%), and laparoscopic colectomy (24 cases, 6%). One hundred and eleven (27%) cases had a laparoscopic approach, and 6 cases (5%) were converted to open surgery. Ten complications (2%) were reported (liver bleeding, trocar port bleeding, bile collection, postoperative ileus, wound infection, serosal tears, iliac artery rupture). Three surveys were not reporting any clinical outcomes and are not included in the table.

Abbreviations: UH university hospital, *Lap* laparoscopic, *NA* no information

Table 9.2 Surgical telementoring surveys with an educational primary outcome

Educational aspects		Specifications ($n=7$)
Mentors		7
Participants	Medical students	63
	Surgical residents	24
	General surgeons	48
Procedures (number of surveys n)		Laparoscopic cholecystectomy (1)
		Bovine surgery (2)
		Endoscopic procedures (1)
		Open thyroidectomy (1)
Educational outcome (number of surveys n)		Global Operative Assessment of Laparoscopic Skills (1)
		Global Rating Scale (1)
		Recognition anatomical landmarks (3)
		Task performance (navigation, clip applying, grasping, suturing, economy of movement) (2)
Simulators		2
Robotics		3
Stationary VC units		5
Mobile VC units		2
In-house VC		4
Cross-institutional VC		3
Intercontinental VC		2
Improved surgical achievement		7

All surveys in the review (27) had some form of educational aspects in their discussion; however, only seven surveys (27%) reported a primary outcome focusing on education. All of these surveys report improved surgical achievement

Discussion

Findings Summary

Present understanding of the effects of videoconference technology on surgical practice is limited. Three hundred and ninety-two surgical procedures were reported, with a complication frequency of 4%. This complication frequency is comparable to on-site surgery. Laparoscopic cholecystectomy, colectomy, and endovascular treatment of aortic aneurysm were the most common procedures. All surveys focus on education; however, only seven surveys (27%) have a systematic evaluation of surgical performance and educational outcome. Most surveys were either cross institutional or between countries; perceived usefulness of surgical telementoring was high among 83% of surgical trainees. There is considerable room for improvement of research quality, as only 27% of the papers had defined a clear research question. Similarly, only 30% of the surveys performed an evaluation of user satisfaction of the technological solution.

Table 9.3 Technical features of telementoring equipment 2000–2010

Technical feature		Setting		
		Experimental/simulation (n=10)	Clinical (n=17)	Overall n=27 (%)
Choice of technical solution (missing 4)	Commercial	6	12	18 (66)
	In-house	3	0	3 (11)
	Freeware	1	1	2 (7)
Bandwidth[a] (missing 8)	<150 k	1	1	2 (7)
	150–512 k	7	8	15 (58)
	768 k–1.2 m–54 m	1	4	5 (18)
Video encoding (missing 17)	H 261–263	2	3	5 (18)
	H 320–323	2	0	2 (7)
	MPEG4	2	0	2 (7)
Resolution (missing 18)	176×144	3	1	4 (15)
	320×240	2	2	4 (15)
	344×288			
	768×492	1	0	1 (4)
	1,024×768			
Delay (ms)[b] (missing 18)	<100	1	0	1 (4)
	100–500	0	5	5 (18)
	>500	2	0	2 (7)
Equipment	Mobile	5	0	5 (18)
	Telestration	4	8	12 (44)
	Telepresence robot	1	2	3 (11)
Organization of telementor service	In-house	5	5	10 (38)
	Cross institutional	3	13	16 (59)
	Intracountry	7	9	16 (59)
	Intercountry	2	6	8 (29)
	Intercontinental			

Five studies report some technical problems, while 10 studies report no technical problems. The rest of surveys do not report information about technical problems

Definitions: Clinical study: study performed in a real clinical setting transferring live video; experimental/simulation study: other studies

Abbreviations: kbps=kilobytes per second (k); Mbps=megabytes per second (m), *ms* milliseconds

[a] Bandwidth: is a measure of available or consumed data communication resources expressed in bits/second or multiples of it (kilobits/s, megabits/s etc.)

[b] Delay: video transmission delay

Clinical Aspects

Recently, a meta-analysis supports evidence that trainees can obtain similar clinical results to expert surgeons in laparoscopic colorectal surgery if supervised by an experienced trainer [6]. Two surveys of laparoscopic telementoring [43, 45] were included in this review, showing no significant difference in conversion, anastomotic leak, or mortality compared to on-site mentoring. Similar results were also shown by Panait et al. [38]. In our review, there is a 2% overall complication rate and 6% conversion rate, which is in accordance with other surveys [6]. One study reports decreased operation time of telementoring [32] compared to physical presence. In contrast, Schlachta's [42, 43] surveys revealed an increased operating time, but a significant decrease in hospital days. Most studies were neither randomized nor controlled, and this makes it difficult to estimate the significance of the findings. Some studies made references to literature [29, 53] for control purposes, while most merely reported absolute figures [8, 30, 31, 37, 45, 49]. There is no evidence in included studies of increased cost-effectiveness of surgical telementoring, for instance, reduced transfers between hospitals or other terms of resource utilization.

Education of Surgeons

Unless the rate at which general surgeons are trained increases, the number of general surgeons per population will continue to decline [54]. In 2003, Etzioni et al. [55, 56] found that, as a result of an expanding/aging population, there would be a 31% increase in surgical work between 2001 and 2020. More recently, Williams et al. [57] estimated that, in 2030, there would be a 9% shortage in the general surgical workforce, with greater shortages in other surgical specialties. This means that rate and volume of surgical education has to increase; videoconference and telementoring can be used to meet this demand. Telementoring as a tool for education between different levels of health care has been described by different surgical subspecialities [58, 59]. Demartines et al. [60, 61] assessed telemedicine in surgical education and patient care. Seventy teleconferences were held, participant satisfaction was high, transmission of clinical documents was accurate, and the opportunity to discuss case management significantly improved. However, bringing together multiple experts to focus, as a group, on a single patient is an organizational and logistical challenge. With VC and telementoring, discussion of a series of patients among a broad range of experts is possible across vast distances, resulting in a level of consultation at a cost otherwise not possible.

VC is widely used for educational purposes for surgeons throughout the world. The rapid evolution of scientific and technical knowledge in surgery explains the demand by surgeons and surgical students for easy and full access to high-quality information. In remote areas, VC has been proven to be an effective educational tool. An Australian study provided synchronous tutorials in pediatric surgery using VC at two rural sites with the tutor located at a metropolitan pediatric clinical school. VC surgical tutorials were highly valued by graduate medical students as an educational method [62]. Similarly, a successful educational VC project was recently reported from Africa, where the shortage of pediatric surgeons is acute [63]. Telementoring is an effective method for didactic lectures in a surgical clerkship. This technology allows students to receive interactive lectures at remote clinical sites without the need to travel over long distances [64].

User and Mentor Aspects

One major aspect in achieving adoption of new technology and training methods is the experience of the mentors and trainees. Our review shows that evidence of user acceptance of current technology is lacking. Some studies focus on the mentors' and trainees' satisfaction with the technological solution used for telementoring [32, 35, 38, 46–48]. Of these studies, both Sereno and Schneider report medium-perceived picture quality. As only Schneider reports resolution of video, no evidence from systematic studies therefore exists on what picture resolution is required to achieve high-perceived video resolution quality among mentors and trainees. In the evaluation of perceived audio quality, the studies report high-perceived quality in 60% of the studies. Again, the systematic studies report medium-perceived audio quality. Another important user aspect is experienced delay. Few studies (10) report measured delay, and very few reports how the delay was measured (both ways vs. only one way). We used an acceptance criterion of 250 ms, one way, and 500 ms, both ways, based on our experience with videoconferencing and when the communication delay hampers communication.

Technological Aspects

From a technological perspective, aspects like video encoding and video resolution in telementoring solutions are important. Video encoding affects, for instance, how nuances in color of the intestines get represented in the video signal. Picture resolution affects what anatomical landmarks may be identified with a high degree of certainty. It is therefore surprising that these two aspects are the least reported; only three studies report the video resolution used and at the same time provides an evaluation of perceived picture quality. A video resolution of 768×492 and higher is perceived to give high-perceived video quality, while 320×240 and lower is evaluated to provide medium-perceived picture quality. Of other important technical aspects is the ability for the mentor to use telestration. This is the most reported technical feature, and it seems like this feature is mandatory for all telementoring solutions.

Future Technology Perspectives

The current focus on mobile devices such as cell phones and tablet PCs opens a new research dimension. There has been renewed interest in mobile telemedicine solutions owing to new and emerging mobile technology such as third and fourth generation of mobile device communication (3 G and 4 G), increased usability of mobile phones, and Internet-enabled mobile devices.

VC as a clinical tool has been used in multiple settings during the past decades [18]; however, most of these systems have been stationary units. A mobile videoconference solution will bring new and important aspects to this technology, as surgeons can transport and use the system in multiple settings. The impact of this new and emerging technology on surgery collaboration is not easy to determine because the potential effects have not previously been studied in detail. We believe that mobile videoconference solutions based on iPad technology have a potential to positively impact medical practice, especially in rural areas. Research on mobile devices in health-care settings is emerging, with many unsolved issues and potential for exciting new discoveries.

Future Telementor Research

Most studies included in this review were classified as Friedman's phase III (80% system installation) and were designed as prospective observational surveys. In our opinion, the phase for small prospective telementor trials is over, and investigational trials must be replaced with larger systematic trials. Technological barriers (at least in the Western world) to VC have been substantially reduced, and high-quality commercial solutions for telementoring and VC are easy accessible. There is therefore less need for surveys focusing on technical aspects. In our opinion, future telementor trials must increase focus on:

- *Education of surgeons*: There is a large demand in society for new surgeons. How can VC and telementoring contribute to a more cost-effective education?
- *Clinical aspects*: Is telementoring a safe method to educate new or inexperienced surgeons or do complication rates increase when surgical education is not performed hands-on?
- *Telementoring in combination with emerging technology*: How can telementoring be combined with simulators, robotics, and mobile platforms for educational and clinical purposes?
- *Licensure and liability problems*: Telementoring is often performed across organizational borders. Expert surgeons at university hospitals usually have an extremely tight schedule with no extra time to mentor surgeons at a local hospital. How shall organizational issues like licensure, credentialing, hospital finances, legal matters, and potential malpractice be dealt with?

Conclusion

Our experiences as well as a comprehensive review of the medical literature [26], shows that surgical telementoring is well suited for surgical training and education. However, implementation of telemedicine and videoconference is slower than expected within the surgical community. Technological barriers to surgical telementoring have decreased during recent years, and high-quality videoconference equipment is accessible on a commercial basis. Our previous review [26] assessing more than 392 surgical procedures when compared to on-site mentoring. To meet the increasing demand for general surgeons, surgical telementoring for educational purposes should be further explored and evaluated. New surgical telementor surveys should have clearly defined research objectives, assessing clinical and educational aspects in a systematic manner.

References

1. Aucar JA, Doarn CR, Sargsyan A, Samuelson DA, Odonnell MJ, DeBakey ME. Use of the Internet for long-term clinical follow-up. Telemed J. 1998;4(4):371–4.
2. DeBakey ME. Telemedicine has now come of age. Telemed J. 1995;1(1):3–4.
3. Merrell RC, Doarn CR. In Memoriam Michael E. DeBakey, MD. 1908–2008. Telemed J E Health. 2008;14(6):503–4.
4. Jarvis-Selinger S, Chan E, Payne R, Plohman K, Ho K. Clinical telehealth across the disciplines: lessons learned. Telemed J E Health. 2008;14(7):720–5.
5. Doarn CR. The power of video conferencing in surgical practice and education. World J Surg. 2009;33(7):1366–7.
6. Miskovic D, Wyles SM, Ni M, Darzi AW, Hanna GB. Systematic review on mentoring and simulation in laparoscopic colorectal surgery. Ann Surg. 2010;252(6):943–51.
7. Doarn CR. Telemedicine in tomorrow's operating room: a natural fit. Semin Laparosc Surg. 2003;10(3):121–6.
8. Rothenberg SS, Yoder S, Kay S, Ponsky T. Initial experience with surgical telementoring in pediatric laparoscopic surgery using remote presence technology. J Laparoendosc Adv Surg Tech A. 2009;19 Suppl 1:S219–22.
9. Damore LJ, Johnson JA, Dixon RS, Iverson MA, Ellison EC, Melvin WS. Transmission of live laparoscopic surgery over the Internet2. Am J Surg. 1999;178(5):415–7.
10. Matsumoto E, Lee L, Warren J, Caumartin Y, Shetty A, Touma N, et al. Long-distance telementoring: prospective trial in training laparoscopic radical prostatectomy. J Urol. 2009;181 (4, Supplement 1):822–3.
11. Agarwal R, Levinson AW, Allaf M, Markov D, Nason A, Su LM. The RoboConsultant: telementoring and remote presence in the operating room during minimally invasive urologic surgeries using a novel mobile robotic interface. Urology. 2007;70(5):970–4.
12. Anvari M. Telesurgery: remote knowledge translation in clinical surgery. World J Surg. 2007; 31(8):1545–50.
13. Ballantyne GH. Robotic surgery, telerobotic surgery, telepresence, and telementoring. Review of early clinical results. Surg Endosc. 2002;16(10).1389–402.
14. Augestad KM, Lindsetmo RO. Overcoming distance: video-conferencing as a clinical and educational tool among surgeons. World J Surg. 2009;33(7):1356–65.
15. Merrell RC, Doarn CR. Is it time for a telemedicine breakthrough? Telemed J E Health. 2008; 14(6):505–6.
16. Lim EC, Seet RC. In-house medical education: redefining tele-education. Teach Learn Med. 2008;20(2):193–5.
17. Dickson-Witmer D, Petrelli NJ, Witmer DR, England M, Witkin G, Manzone T, et al. A statewide community cancer center videoconferencing program. Ann Surg Oncol. 2008;15(11): 3058–64.
18. Wood D. No surgeon should operate alone: how telementoring could change operations. Telemed J E Health. 2011;17(3):150–2.
19. Friedman CP. Where's the science in medical informatics? J Am Med Inform Assoc. 1995; 2(1):65–7.
20. Vuolio S, Winblad I, Ohinmaa A, Haukipuro K. Videoconferencing for orthopaedic outpatients: one-year follow-up. J Telemed Telecare. 2003;9(1):8–11.
21. Wallace P, Haines A, Harrison R, Barber J, Thompson S, Jacklin P, et al. Joint teleconsultations (virtual outreach) versus standard outpatient appointments for patients referred by their general practitioner for a specialist opinion: a randomised trial. Lancet. 2002;359(9322): 1961–8.
22. Ohinmaa A, Vuolio S, Haukipuro K, Winblad I. A cost-minimization analysis of orthopaedic consultations using videoconferencing in comparison with conventional consulting. J Telemed Telecare. 2002;8(5):283–9.

23. Camara JG, Zabala RR, Henson RD, Senft SH. Teleophthalmology: the use of real-time tele-mentoring to remove an orbital tumor. Ophthalmology. 2000;107(8):1468–71.
24. Schulam PG, Docimo SG, Saleh W, Breitenbach C, Moore RG, Kavoussi L. Telesurgical mentoring. Initial clinical experience. Surg Endosc. 1997;11(10):1001–5.
25. Rosser JC, Wood M, Payne JH, Fullum TM, Lisehora GB, Rosser LE, et al. Telementoring. A practical option in surgical training. Surg Endosc. 1997;11(8):852–5.
26. Augestad KM, Chomutare T, Bellika G, Patel HRH, Lindsetmo RO, Delaney CP, Mobile Medical Mentor Group (M3). Education of Surgeons and Risk of Complications During Surgical Telemetoring. Surgical Innovation 2011.
27. Rodas EB, Latifi R, Cone S, Broderick TJ, Doarn CR, Merrell RC. Telesurgical presence and consultation for open surgery. Arch Surg. 2002;137(12):1360–3; discussion 1363.
28. Bauer J. International surgical telementoring using a robotic arm: our experience. Telemed J. 2000;6(1):25–31.
29. Bruschi M, Micali S, Porpiglia F, Celia A, De Stefani S, Grande M, et al. Laparoscopic tele-mentored adrenalectomy: the Italian experience. Surg Endosc. 2005;19(6):836–40.
30. Byrne JP, Mughal MM. Telementoring as an adjunct to training and competence-based assess-ment in laparoscopic cholecystectomy. Surg Endosc. 2000;14(12):1159–61.
31. Challacombe B, Kandaswamy R, Dasgupta P, Mamode N. Telementoring facilitates indepen-dent hand-assisted laparoscopic living donor nephrectomy. Transplant Proc. 2005;37(2):613–6.
32. Ereso AQ, Garcia P, Tseng E, Gauger G, Kim H, Dua MM, et al. Live transference of surgical subspecialty skills using telerobotic proctoring to remote general surgeons. J Am Coll Surg. 2010;211(3):400–11.
33. Ewers R, Schicho K, Wagner A, Undt G, Seemann R, Figl M, et al. Seven years of clinical experience with teleconsultation in craniomaxillofacial surgery. J Oral Maxillofac Surg. 2005;63(10):1447–54.
34. Gambadauro P, Magos A. NEST (network enhanced surgical training): a PC-based system for telementoring in gynaecological surgery. Eur J Obstet Gynecol Reprod Biol. 2008;139(2):222–5.
35. Gandsas A, McIntire K, Montgomery K, Bumgardner C, Rice L. The personal digital assistant (PDA) as a tool for telementoring endoscopic procedures. Stud Health Technol Inform. 2004;98:99–103.
36. Mendez I, Hill R, Clarke D, Kolyvas G. Robotic long-distance telementoring in neurosurgery. Neurosurgery. 2005;56(3):434–40; discussion 434–40.
37. Rodrigues Netto Jr N, Mitre AI, Lima SV, Fugita OE, Lima ML, Stoianovici D, et al. Telementoring between Brazil and the United States: initial experience. J Endourol. 2003;17(4):217–20.
38. Panait L, Rafiq A, Tomulescu V, Boanca C, Popescu I, Carbonell A, et al. Telementoring versus on-site mentoring in virtual reality-based surgical training. Surg Endosc. 2006;20(1):113–8.
39. Rafiq A, Moore JA, Zhao X, Doarn CR, Merrell RC. Digital video capture and synchronous consultation in open surgery. Ann Surg. 2004;239(4):567–73.
40. Schlachta CM, Mamazza J, Seshadri PA, Cadeddu M, Gregoire R, Poulin EC. Defining a learning curve for laparoscopic colorectal resections. Dis Colon Rectum. 2001;44(2):217–22.
41. Sawyer MA, Lim RB, Wong SY, Cirangle PT, Birkmire-Peters D. Telementored laparoscopic cholecystectomy: a pilot study. Stud Health Technol Inform. 2000;70:302–8.
42. Schlachta CM, Lefebvre KL, Sorsdahl AK, Jayaraman S. Mentoring and telementoring leads to effective incorporation of laparoscopic colon surgery. Surg Endosc. 2010;24(4):841–4.
43. Schlachta CM, Sorsdahl AK, Lefebvre KL, McCune ML, Jayaraman S. A model for longitu-dinal mentoring and telementoring of laparoscopic colon surgery. Surg Endosc. 2009;23(7):1634–8.
44. Sebajang H, Trudeau P, Dougall A, Hegge S, McKinley C, Anvari M. Telementoring: an important enabling tool for the community surgeon. Surg Innov. 2005;12(4):327–31.
45. Sebajang H, Trudeau P, Dougall A, Hegge S, McKinley C, Anvari M. The role of telementor-ing and telerobotic assistance in the provision of laparoscopic colorectal surgery in rural areas. Surg Endosc. 2006;20(9):1389–93.

46. Schneider A, Wilhelm D, Doll D, Rauschenbach U, Finkenzeller M, Wirnhier H, et al. Wireless live streaming video of surgical operations: an evaluation of communication quality. J Telemed Telecare. 2007;13(8):391–6.
47. Sereno S, Mutter D, Dallemagne B, Smith CD, Marescaux J. Telementoring for minimally invasive surgical training by wireless robot. Surg Innov. 2007;14(3):184–91.
48. Snyder CW, Vandromme MJ, Tyra SL, Hawn MT. Proficiency-based laparoscopic and endoscopic training with virtual reality simulators: a comparison of proctored and independent approaches. J Surg Educ. 2009;66(4):201–7.
49. Tamariz F, Merrell R, Popescu I, Onisor D, Flerov Y, Boanca C, et al. Design and implementation of a web-based system for intraoperative consultation. World J Surg. 2009;33(3):448–54.
50. Di Valentino M, Alerci M, Bogen M, Tutta P, Sartori F, Marty B, et al. Telementoring during endovascular treatment of abdominal aortic aneurysms: a prospective study. J Endovasc Ther. 2005;12(2):200–5.
51. Parker A, Rubinfeld I, Azuh O, Blyden D, Falvo A, Horst M, et al. What ring tone should be used for patient safety? Early results with a Blackberry-based telementoring safety solution. Am J Surg. 2010;199(3):336–40; discussion 340–1.
52. Seemann R, Guevara G, Undt G, Ewers R, Schicho K. Clinical evaluation of tele-endoscopy using UMTS cellphones. Surg Endosc. 2010;24(11):2855–9.
53. Bauer JJ, Lee BR, Stoianovici D, Bishoff JT, O'Kelley S, Cadeddu JA, et al. Remote Telesurgical Mentoring: Feasibility and Efficacy. Proceedings of the 33rd Hawaii International Conference on System Sciences-Volume 5—Volume 5: IEEE Computer Society, 2000.
54. Etzioni DA, Finlayson SR, Ricketts TC, Lynge DC, Dimick JB. Getting the science right on the surgeon workforce issue. Arch Surg. 2011;146(4):381–4.
55. Etzioni DA, Liu JH, O'Connell JB, Maggard MA, Ko CY. Elderly patients in surgical workloads: a population-based analysis. Am Surg. 2003;69(11):961–5.
56. Etzioni DA, Liu JH, Maggard MA, Ko CY. The aging population and its impact on the surgery workforce. Ann Surg. 2003;238(2):170–7.
57. Williams Jr TE, Satiani B, Thomas A, Ellison EC. The impending shortage and the estimated cost of training the future surgical workforce. Ann Surg. 2009;250(4):590–7.
58. Demartines N, Mutter D, Marescaux J, Harder F. Preliminary assessment of the value and effect of expert consultation in telemedicine. J Am Coll Surg. 2000;190(4):466–70.
59. Fleissig A, Jenkins V, Catt S, Fallowfield L. Multidisciplinary teams in cancer care: are they effective in the UK? Lancet Oncol. 2006;7(11):935–43.
60. Demartines N, Mutter D, Vix M, Leroy J, Glatz D, Rosel F, et al. Assessment of telemedicine in surgical education and patient care. Ann Surg. 2000;231(2):282–91.
61. Demartines N, Otto U, Mutter D, Labler L, von Weymarn A, Vix M, et al. An evaluation of telemedicine in surgery: telediagnosis compared with direct diagnosis. Arch Surg. 2000;135(7):849–53.
62. Holland AJ, Soundappan SV, Oldmeadow W. Videoconferencing surgical tutorials: bridging the gap. ANZ J Surg. 2008;78(4):297–301.
63. Hadley GP, Mars M. Postgraduate medical education in paediatric surgery: videoconferencing – a possible solution for Africa? Pediatr Surg Int. 2008;24(2):223–6.
64. Stain SC, Mitchell M, Belue R, Mosley V, Wherry S, Adams CZ, et al. Objective assessment of videoconferenced lectures in a surgical clerkship. Am J Surg. 2005;189(1):81–4.

Chapter 10
Portable Learning and Multimedia in Surgical Training

Narinderjit Singh Kullar, Stig Müller, and Hitendra R.H. Patel

Abstract Instructional methods that aim to optimize teaching outside of the operating room are becoming increasingly important due to the reduction in traditional hospital training hours. One such method is the use of multimedia-based portable learning tools. In developing these tools, due consideration should be given to the features that define effective multimedia and the core surgical skills suited to this form of instruction.

Multimedia is effective for both technical and nontechnical surgical skills acquisition either in isolation or as an adjunct to other methods. The key proficiencies to which multimedia instruction is suited include factual and theoretical knowledge, intraoperative decision-making, and error identification. In addition, such applications can also be used as an adjunct to other methods for the purpose of dexterity, visual-spatial ability, and perceptual skills development.

The principles of effective multimedia design include an engaging interface with ease of navigation, employing the use of interactivity to promote active learning, methods for assessment and feedback, and most importantly, the inclusion of well-scripted video material, still imagery, and animation with on-screen text kept to a minimum.

The use of multimedia learning tools for surgical skills development is becoming increasingly important. This form of instruction is able to facilitate the acquisition of several core technical and nontechnical skills in an effective manner provided due consideration is given to the principles of effective multimedia design.

N.S. Kullar, MBBS, M.Sc.(MedEd), MRCS • S. Müller, M.D., Ph.D.
H.R.H. Patel, MD, PhD (✉)
Department of Urology and Endocrine Surgery,
University Hospital North Norway,
Breivika, Tromsø N-9038, Norway
e-mail: hrhpatel@hotmail.com

H.R.H. Patel, J.V. Joseph (eds.), *Simulation Training in Laparoscopy and Robotic Surgery*,
DOI 10.1007/978-1-4471-2930-1_10, © Springer-Verlag London 2012

Keywords Surgical training • Competency • Portable learning • Multimedia Virtual reality

Key Points
- Portable multimedia applications are becoming increasingly important for surgical skills training.
- Surgical skill comprises both technical and nontechnical components which should be reflected in the content and design of multimedia applications.
- Multimedia instruction is particularly suited to the development of factual and theoretical knowledge, intraoperative decision-making, and error identification.
- Multimedia is also of value as an adjunct to other instructional methods for the purpose of dexterity, visual-spatial ability, and perceptual skills development.
- Interpersonal skills are difficult to develop through the use of multimedia but multimedia is better suited for simulation-based training.
- The multimedia interface should be engaged to maintain the interest of the viewer, with simple means of navigation between differing instructional elements.
- Video material should be deconstructed into the constituent steps of the procedure identified by cognitive task analysis in order to aid development of cognitive skills such as decision-making.
- Graphical elements should promote learning and should not be included for aesthetic purposes. In using animation and still imagery, key views with minor degrees of rotation are preferable to interactive 3-D modeling.
- Narrative should be well scripted and synchronized to video elements with principles such as cueing employed to facilitate learning with on-screen text kept to a minimum.
- Methods for feedback and pre- and posttesting of trainees should be included to guide goal development and goal reflection, respectively.

Introduction

Increasing accountability for patient safety and medical errors along with the greater complexity of surgical procedures has resulted in fewer opportunities for training [1]. Changing work patterns, with an increasing reliance on shift systems and a reduction in both work and training hours, have further compounded the problems of training provision. Surgical trainees are increasingly finding themselves removed from normal working hours during which the majority of traditional operative training and experience is gained [2]. The deleterious effects of this reduced operative exposure have fuelled the development of alternative instructional methods to optimize teaching outside of the operating room, the most notable of which are the use of simulation and multimedia.

Instructional multimedia can be defined as the integration of text, images (both still and moving), and sound within a single educational medium [3]. In line with improving technology, there has been increasing use of these portable learning tools from the use of CD-ROM, DVD, and Blu-ray through to online streaming to desktops and the recent growth in mobile Internet. The use of portable multimedia is already widespread in surgical education and is likely to be increasingly important given the reduction of in-hospital training hours. In the context of surgical skills acquisition, the use of multimedia-based instruction should go beyond the simple demonstration of surgical technique by means of footage captured during a procedure. It is well recognized that the successful outcome of a complex surgical procedure is multifaceted and dependent on other nontechnical factors in addition to technical [4–6]. While simulation-based training is evolving to incorporate teaching of nontechnical skills, multimedia applications have thus far tended to concentrate on technical skills learning in isolation. The importance of nontechnical skills cannot be underestimated, with communication failures alone accounting for almost half of the causal factors that lead to errors in surgery [6]. Furthermore, it has been reported that a surgical procedure is 75% cognitive skill and 25% technical [7]. However, it is possible to incorporate instruction in many nontechnical areas through a considered approach to multimedia design and structure.

Multimedia and Surgical Skills

In developing multimedia-based tools for operative training, it is valuable to initially consider these constituent skills which collectively define operative competence. An understanding of the proficiencies to which multimedia training is suited in combination with intelligent interface design is an essential prerequisite when constructing effective applications. The component elements of operative competence are summarized in Fig. 10.1 and comprise both technical and nontechnical skills.

The key technical components appear to be visual-spatial ability, perceptual skill, and psychomotor skill, which itself is a combination of knowledge and dexterity [4, 7, 8]. Importantly, while visual-spatial skill appears to be a key innate attribute, the consensus opinion among expert surgeons both in the United Kingdom and worldwide was that the important operative skills required of a competent surgeon or trainee were generic ability relating to tissue handling (psychomotor) and correct contextual use of dangerous instrumentation (perceptual) [9, 10].

Visual-spatial ability is an innate attribute, which correlates with the ability to learn a new task [8]. Despite this, poor visual-spatial ability can be overcome through additional practice and feedback [8]. While it would appear that multimedia has little direct role in developing visual-spatial ability, demonstration of key views

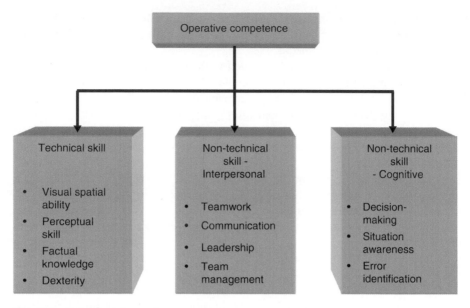

Fig. 10.1 Algorithm of operative competence

by means of animation can assist trainees with poor visual-spatial ability overcome difficulties in learning spatial tasks [11, 12].

Perceptual skill is a function of both experience and judgment of a given circumstance or operative context and should not be confused with depth perception, which is an innate attribute similar to visual-spatial ability [4, 13]. This type of skill is primarily acquired through experience gained in the operating room but could be supported by multimedia applications that include multiple operative context of the same procedure.

Multimedia has been shown to be particularly effective in developing operative dexterity either in isolation or in conjunction with other instructional methods. In isolation, multimedia training has been shown to be of value in improving actual performance [14]. In addition, it has also been shown to be superior to print media regardless of the level of interactivity employed [15]. The combination of multimedia with other instructional methods increases the effectiveness further, particularly when group multimedia instruction is followed by individual practice using simulated tissue [16]. Educational techniques involving cognitive frameworks, such as cognitive task analysis (CTA), increase the efficacy still further [14, 17]. Such cognitive methods aim to delineate not only the individual steps involved but also the sensory cues and higher thought processes that occur during the course of a complex procedure. This form of instruction has an additional benefit of not requiring an expert to facilitate learning and is ideally suited to portable learning methods.

In terms of theoretical knowledge, multimedia is as effective as print medium and standard lectures but has been shown to be superior when applying such knowledge to the operating room/theater [15, 18, 19]. Again, incorporation of CTA principles can further improve the efficacy in terms of both the immediate understanding of the procedure and the subsequent retention of knowledge [20]. From a student's perspective, web-based multimedia exercises have been found to be highly accessible, easy to use, engaging, and realistic, with a high degree of reported satisfaction and motivation to learn [21–23]. Furthermore, a greater proportion of learners are reported to prefer the use of a computer as the primary source of information when compared to expert tutoring [21]. An important aspect within this domain is knowledge of anatomy and anatomical plane recognition. For this purpose, multimedia instruction is sufficient as a stand-alone tool for the purpose of teaching simple anatomy and is perceived by trainees as being superior to traditional methods [24, 25].

Nontechnical skills can be divided into those relating to interpersonal characteristics and cognitive functioning. In terms of interpersonal qualities required, teamwork and communication are of prime importance [4–7, 26, 27]. Other important nontechnical interpersonal skills include leadership, team management, and to a lesser extent planning and preparation [5, 6]. The important cognitive skills are decision-making ability, situation awareness, and error identification [5–7, 26]. Lesser cognitive skills include risk assessment, anticipation, and adaption [6].

Interpersonal skills are primarily developed during the course of actual procedures and daily surgical practice. Simulated environments utilizing anesthetists, surgeons, and nursing staff appear to show the most promise in developing interpersonal skills outside of the operating room [27, 28]. With improving technology, it may be possible to produce an interactive application akin to simulation that addresses issues related to interpersonal training; however, at present, the effectiveness of multimedia in this domain is limited.

In contrast to the ineffectual role played by multimedia instruction for interpersonal skills acquisition, multimedia technology appears to have greater significance in the context of cognitive skills training. This was initially noted in a comparative study of multimedia and conventional training for general cognitive surgical skills development [29]. The outcome of this early study found that multimedia instruction brought all groups of learners to a comparable level of cognitive knowledge regardless of prior experience. Of the constituent components that together comprise cognitive nontechnical skills, decision-making appears to be the area in which multimedia has the greatest potential.

The importance of operative decision-making should not be underestimated; it has been suggested that of the important events during an operation, 75% relate to decision-making ability with the remainder relating to technique [30]. Digital multimedia has proven benefit in improving individual decision-making skills, particularly when CTA principles are applied [14, 31, 32]. The use of web-based multimedia has similarly been shown to lead to improvement in this skill and has the additional benefit of high levels of user friendliness [22, 23]. Finally, multimedia has also been shown to be of partial benefit in developing team-based problem solving [19].

The ability to identify errors has been correlated with procedural performance and is an important cognitive skill [33]. It would appear relatively simple to incorporate error identification within a multimedia platform perhaps as part of an interactive formative exercise utilizing video and animation.

The final skill is situation awareness, which refers to noticing, understanding, and predicting the important features of a dynamic environment [26]. Given the nature of this trait however, multimedia training is unlikely to be of benefit.

Multimedia Design and Structure

The essential components of effective multimedia design relate to interface design, interactivity, the use of video and still imagery, animation, narrative, and assessment and feedback. It should be noted that in designing applications, each of these should merit equal consideration. The key features of the core areas are summarized in Table 10.1.

An approachable, user-friendly interface is perceived as one of the key benefits to learners [19, 22, 23]. Of note, navigation should be simple and require low mental effort in line with cognitive load theory [34–36]. The navigation framework should also allow easy access to material appropriate for all user levels, perhaps with supplementary hyperlinks for access to further resources [25, 34]. Also, the interface should be sufficiently engaging so as to maintain the interest of the learner and promote interactivity [37]. Junior trainees should be guided through a complete procedure for orientation by limiting the degree of navigation [34]. In contrast, the medium should also allow senior trainees to navigate to those parts of a procedure that are of greatest relevance to their educational needs, as per adult learning theory [38]. The navigational framework could also be extended via the use of supplementary hyperlinks for access to other resources [25].

Interactivity is essential and engenders true active learning if you accept that students retain 20% of what they hear, 40% of what they see, and 75% of what they see, hear, and interact with [34, 39]. However, some studies suggest that the inclusion of interactivity leads to no improvement over and above standard noninteractive multimedia [18, 40]. However, it is also noted that this tends to be the case for simple tasks only [18, 40]. For the purpose of more complex operations, the evidence for including a degree of interactivity appears logical and suggests that a degree of interactivity is important.

In presenting video material, it is crucial that all footage is authentic with redundant material excluded [34]. Adults tend to learn in areas of greatest relevance [38]. To encourage this aspect of adult learning theory, video material should be presented as a series of procedural steps, identified by CTA, with individual clips accessible via the navigational framework [14, 31, 32]. For each step of the procedure, the inclusion of multiple video clips from differing operative context would facilitate teaching of important cognitive skills such as decision-making [14, 20]. The platform should also be updated on a regular basis to allow for dissemination of newer techniques [41].

The incorporation of animation and still imagery is also beneficial and should be included as part of a multilevel approach to media design [29]. The use of still imagery and 3-D animation are especially suited to anatomy instruction, a key aspect of operative

Table 10.1 Recommended multimedia design features

Media component	Recommended design
Interface	The interface should be engaged to maintain the interest of the viewer, with simple means of navigation between differing instructional elements. Navigation should be relatively restricted for junior trainees with greater freedom afforded to senior learners. Supplementary material should be made accessible via the application
Video material	Video material should be deconstructed into the constituent steps of the procedure identified by cognitive task analysis. Consider including multiple examples of each step to demonstrate aspects relating to cognitive skills such as decision-making
Graphics	Graphical elements should promote learning and not be used for aesthetic purposes only. In using animation and still imagery, key views with minor degrees of rotation should be used in preference to interactive 3-D modeling
Narrative	Narrative should be well scripted and synchronized to video elements. Principles such as cueing should be used to facilitate learning while on-screen text should be kept to a minimum
Assessment	Methods for pre- and posttesting of trainees should be included to guide goal development and goal reflection, respectively. Feedback of scores should be prompt

surgery in general [11, 12]. When applied to the operative context, the use of 3-D animation in addition to edited video has been found to be more effective in developing anatomical knowledge and recognition skills when compared to video alone [42]. Such animation, however, should be used sparingly in light of the findings that most learners tend to utilize key anatomical views with minor degrees of rotation [11, 12].

According to Mayer [36], "the central work of multimedia learning takes place in working memory." The working memory itself processes information via 2 channels (the visual and the auditory) each of which has a limited capacity for information, or cognitive load. Hence, a well-scripted narrative is equally important as video footage and graphics and should be synchronized to visual elements [34]. Two principles relating to cognitive load act to increase the efficiency of the working memory and are important when considering audio. The first is the "cueing" effect, whereby the relevant areas of an image or video are clearly identified in line with the descriptive audio [36]. The second is the "modality" effect, whereby on-screen text is kept to a minimum by utilizing audio description instead. However, in some instances, a reverse modality effect has also been demonstrated with greatest learning taking place through the use of on-screen text [35]. In accommodating this anomaly, it seems that a minimum of on-screen text should be included along with links to further wording if required.

Assessment exercises should also be given due consideration with both pre- and posttesting of students in order to facilitate goal development and goal reflection, respectively [34]. Such exercises should be formative in nature and should provide immediate focused feedback for the trainee [4, 34, 41, 43].

Conclusion

The use of multimedia training is already widespread and is likely to become increasingly important. To date, such methods have predominantly been used to demonstrate operative principles through the use of video footage captured during surgical procedures. However, the evidence suggests that portable applications have a far wider and significant role in both technical and nontechnical skills acquisition. Surgical skill domains particularly suited to this form of instruction include factual and theoretical knowledge, intraoperative decision-making, and error identification. In addition, such applications can also be used as an adjunct to other methods for the purpose of dexterity, visual-spatial ability, and perceptual skills development.

Finally, the effectiveness of multimedia can be enhanced through a considered approach to design and structure. When developing applications, key areas to address include interface design and navigation, the level of interactivity to be employed, inclusion of appropriate video material, still imagery and animation along with a well-scripted narrative, and methods for assessment and feedback.

References

1. Reznick RK. Surgical simulation. A vital part of our future. Ann Surg. 2005;242(5):640–1.
2. Clarke MD, Anderson ADG, MacFie J. Training the higher surgical trainee within the EWTD framework. Bull R Coll Surg Engl. 2004;86(3):82–4.
3. Reddi UV, Mishra S. Educational multimedia. A handbook for teacher-developers. New Delhi: CEMCA; 2003.
4. Tsue TT, Dugan JW, Burkey B. Assessment of surgical competency. Otolaryngol Clin North Am. 2007;40(6):1237–59.
5. Yule S, Flin R, Paterson-Brown S, Maran N. Non-technical skills for surgeons in the operating room: a review of the literature. Surgery. 2006;139(2):140–9.
6. Yule S, Flin R, Paterson-Brown S, Maran N, Rowley D. Development of a rating system for surgeons' non-technical skills. Med Educ. 2006;40(11):1098–104.
7. Satava RM, Gallagher AG, Pellegrini CA. Surgical competence and surgical proficiency: definitions, taxonomy, and metrics. J Am Coll Surg. 2003;196(6):933–7.
8. Wanzel KR, Hamstra SJ, Anastakis DJ, Matsumoto ED, Cusimano MD. Effect of visual-spatial ability on learning of spatially complex surgical skills. Lancet. 2002;359:230–1.
9. Cuschieri A, Francis N, Crosby J, Hanna GB. What do master surgeons think of surgical competence and revalidation? Am J Surg. 2001;182(2):110–6.
10. Baldwin PJ, Paisley AM, Brown SP. Consultant surgeons' opinion of the skills required of basic surgical trainees. Br J Surg. 1999;86(8):1078–82.
11. Garg AX, Norman G, Sperotable L. How medical students learn spatial anatomy. Lancet. 2001;357:363–4.
12. Garg AX, Norman GR, Eva KW, Sperotable L, Sharan S. Is there any real virtue of virtual reality?: the minor role of multiple orientations in learning anatomy from computers. Acad Med. 2002;77(10 Suppl):S97–9.
13. Stylopoulos N, Vosburgh KG. Assessing technical skill in surgery and endoscopy: a set of metrics and an algorithm (C-PASS) to assess skills in surgical and endoscopic procedures. Surg Innov. 2007;14(2):113–21.

14. Luker KR, Sullivan ME, Peyre SE, Sherman R, Grunwald T. The use of a cognitive task analysis-based multimedia program to teach surgical decision making in flexor tendon repair. Am J Surg. 2008;195(1):11–5.
15. Friedl R, Höppler H, Ecard K, Scholz W, Hannekum A, Oechsner W, Stracke S. Multimedia-driven teaching significantly improves students' performance when compared with a print medium. Ann Thorac Surg. 2006;81(5):1760–6.
16. Kneebone R, ApSimon D. Surgical skills training: simulation and multimedia combined. Med Educ. 2001;35(9):909–15.
17. Velmahos GC, Toutouzas KG, Sillin LF, Chan L, Clark RE, Theodorou D, Maupin F. Cognitive task analysis for teaching technical skills in an inanimate surgical skills laboratory. Am J Surg. 2004;187(1):114–9.
18. Friedl R, Höppler H, Ecard K, Scholz W, Hannekum A, Oechsner W, Stracke S. Comparative evaluation of multimedia driven, interactive, and case-based teaching in heart surgery. Ann Thorac Surg. 2006;82(5):1790–5.
19. Aly M, Elen J, Willems G. Instructional multimedia program versus standard lecture: a comparison of two methods for teaching the undergraduate orthodontic curriculum. Eur J Dent Educ. 2004;8(1):43–6.
20. Sullivan ME, Brown CV, Peyre SE, Salim A, Martin M, Towfigh S, Grunwald T. The use of cognitive task analysis to improve the learning of percutaneous tracheostomy placement. Am J Surg. 2007;193(1):96–9.
21. Corrêa L, de Campos AC, Souza SC, Novelli MD. Teaching oral surgery to undergraduate students: a pilot study using a Web-based practical course. Eur J Dent Educ. 2003;7(3): 111–5.
22. Kalet AL, Coady SH, Hopkins MA, Hochberg MS, Riles TS. Preliminary evaluation of the Web Initiative for Surgical Education (WISE-MD). Am J Surg. 2007;194(1):89–93.
23. Servais EL, Lamorte WW, Agarwal S, Moschetti W, Mallipattu SK, Moulton SL. Teaching surgical decision-making: an interactive, web-based approach. J Surg Res. 2006;134(1):102–6.
24. Inwood MJ, Ahmad J. Development of instructional, interactive, multimedia anatomy dissection software: a student-led initiative. Clin Anat. 2005;18(8):613–7.
25. Schultze-Mosgau S, Zielinski T, Lochner J. Interactive web-based e-lectures with a multimedia online examination. Med Educ. 2004;38(11):1184.
26. Mishra A, Catchpole K, Dale T, McCulloch P. The influence of non-technical performance on technical outcome in laparoscopic cholecystectomy. Surg Endosc. 2008;22(1):68–73.
27. Undre S, Koutantji M, Sevdalis N, Gautama S, Selvapatt N, Williams S, Sains P, McCulloch P, Darzi A, Vincent C. Multidisciplinary crisis simulations: the way forward for training surgical teams. World J Surg. 2007;31(9):1843–53.
28. Marshall RL, Smith JS, Gorman PJ, Krummel TM, Haluck RS, Cooney RN. Use of a human patient simulator in the development of resident trauma management skills. J Trauma. 2001; 51(1):17–21.
29. Rosser JC, Herman B, Risucci DA, Murayama M, Rosser LE, Merrell RC. Effectiveness of a CD-ROM multimedia tutorial in transferring cognitive knowledge essential for laparoscopic skill training. Am J Surg. 2000;179(4):320–4.
30. Spencer CF. Teaching and measuring surgical techniques – the technical evaluation of competence. Bull Am Coll Surg. 1978;63:9–12.
31. Sarker SK, Chang A, Vincent C. Decision making in laparoscopic surgery: a prospective, independent and blinded analysis. Int J Surg. 2008;6(2):98–105.
32. Sarker SK, Rehman S, Ladwa M, Chang A, Vincent C. A decision-making learning and assessment tool in laparoscopic cholecystectomy. Surg Endosc. 2009;23(1):197–203.
33. Bann S, Khan M, Datta V, Darzi A. Surgical skill is predicted by the ability to detect errors. Am J Surg. 2005;189(4):412–5.
34. Grunwald T, Corsbie-Massay C. Guidelines for cognitively efficient multimedia learning tools: educational strategies, cognitive load, and interface design. Acad Med. 2006;81(3): 213–23.

35. Tabbers HK, Martens RL, van Merriënboer JJ. Multimedia instructions and cognitive load theory: effects of modality and cueing. Br J Educ Psychol. 2004;74(1):71–81.
36. Mayer R. Multimedia learning. New York: Cambridge University Press; 2001.
37. Letterie GS. Medical education as a science: the quality of evidence for computer-assisted instruction. Am J Obstet Gynaecol. 2003;188(3):849–53.
38. Knowles MS. The adult learner: a neglected species. 4th ed. Houston: Gulf Publishing; 1990.
39. Amthor GR. Interactive multimedia in education. T H E Jl (Technol Horizons Educ). 1992; 19(2):2–5.
40. Nousiainen M, Brydges R, Backstein D, Dubrowski A. Comparison of expert instruction and computer-based video training in teaching fundamental surgical skills to medical students. Surgery. 2008;143(4):539–44.
41. Mutter D, Bouras G, Marescaux J. Digital technologies and quality improvement in cancer surgery. Eur J Surg Oncol. 2005;31(6):689–94.
42. Prinz A, Bolz M, Findl O. Advantage of three-dimensional animated teaching over traditional surgical videos for teaching ophthalmic surgery: a randomised study. Br J Ophthalmol. 2005;89(11):1495–9.
43. Sidhu RS, Grober ED, Musselman LJ, Reznick RK. Assessing competency in surgery: where to begin? Surgery. 2004;135(1):6–20.

Index

H.R.H. Patel, J.V. Joseph (eds.), *Simulation Training in Laparoscopy and Robotic Surgery*,   101
DOI 10.1007/978-1-4471-2930-1, © Springer-Verlag London 2012

Printed by Printforce, the Netherlands